NUMBER 366

THE ENGLISH EXPERIENCE

ITS RECORD IN EARLY PRINTED BOOKS
PUBLISHED IN FACSIMILE

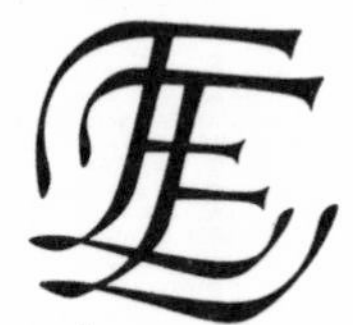

WILLIAM CLOWES

BOOKE OF OBSERVATIONS

LONDON 1596

DA CAPO PRESS
THEATRVM ORBIS TERRARVM LTD.
AMSTERDAM 1971 NEW YORK

The publishers acknowledge their gratitude
to the Syndics of Cambridge University Library
for their permission to reproduce
the Library's copy (Shelfmark: Syn. 7.59.92)
and to the Trustees of the British Museum
for their permission to reproduce
the pages from the Library's copy
(Shelfmark: 7481.d.5.)

Library of Congress Catalog Card Number:
73-171740

S.T.C. No. 5442
Collation: A-Z^4, Aa-Ff^4

Published in 1971 by
Theatrum Orbis Terrarum Ltd.,
O.Z. Voorburgwal 85, Amsterdam
&
Da Capo Press
- a division of Plenum Publishing Corporation -
227 West 17th Street, New York, 10011
Printed in the Netherlands

ISBN 90 221 0366 8

A PROFITABLE AND NECESSARIE Booke of Obſeruations, for all thoſe that are burned with the flame of Gun powder, &c. and alſo for curing of wounds made with Musket and Caliuer ſhot, and other weapons of war commonly vſed at this day both by ſea and land, as heerafter ſhall be declared:

VVith an addition of moſt approoued remedies, gathered for the good and comfort of many, out of diuers learned men both old and new Writers:

Laſt of all is adioined a ſhort Treatiſe, for the cure of *Lues Venerea*, by vnctions and other approoued waies of curing, heertofore by me collected: and now againe newly corrected and augmented in the yeere of our Lorde *1596.*

By WILLIAM CLOWES one of hir Maieſties *Chirurgions.*

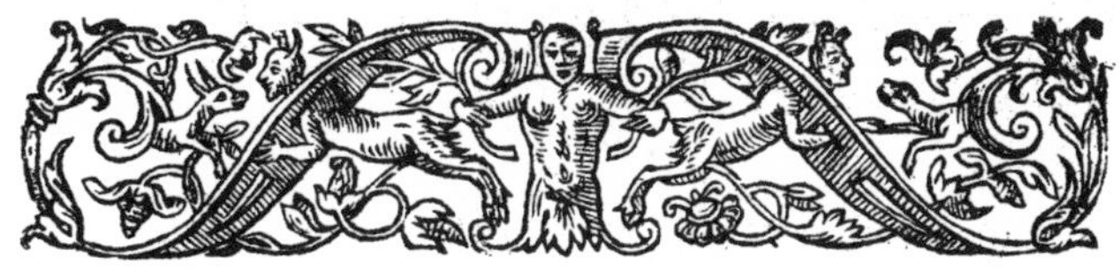

Imprinted at London by Edm. Bollifant, for Thomas Dawſon.

1596

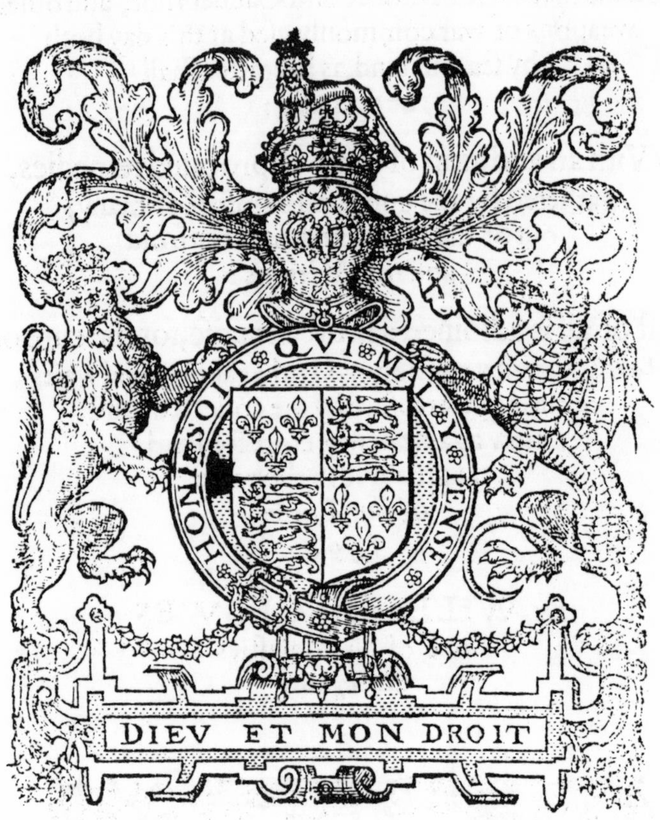
HONI SOIT QVI MAL Y PENSE
DIEV ET MON DROIT

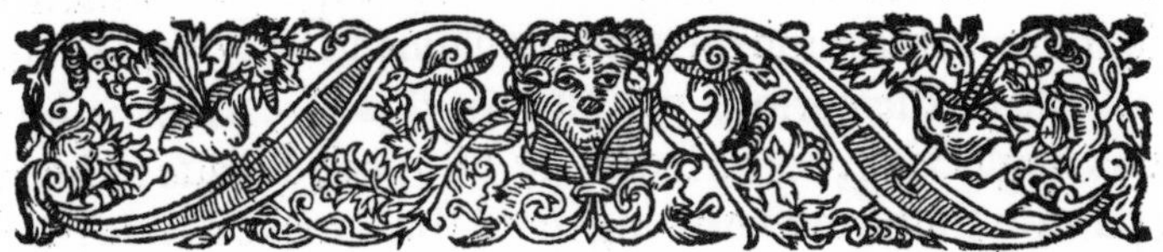

To all the true profeſſors of Chirurgerie in generall whereſoeuer, VVilliam Clowes wiſheth all happines, with much increaſe of knowledge in the art of Chirurgerie.

MOſt louing brethren and friends, vnto you which are ſtudents and practiſers, in the moſt excellent art of Chirurgerie, I do now once againe dedicate this booke, containing diuers ſhort obſeruations of ſome ſpeciall cures by my induſtrious trauell carefully performed, and approoued very profitable for burnings with the flame of Gun powder, and alſo for the curing of wounds made with Musket and Caliuer ſhot, and other weapons of war, commonly vſed at this day both by ſea & land, al which I haue faithfully gathered from diuers reuerend learned Authors, beſides mine owne ſpeciall practiſe: with an addition containing a ſhort treatiſe for the more ſpeedy cure of *Lues Venerea*, now againe newly corrected and augmented, according to my ſeuerall practiſes in theſe yeeres, 1593. 1594. and 1595. the which I leaue to be cenſured by the wiſedomes and iudgements of the learned and diſcreet Readers, not doubting of the great profit, which may ſpeedily growe vnto thoſe, which with a good conſcience ar[illegible]wledge. In which diſcourſe, if I haue for mine owne part chaunced vnawares to ouerſlip my ſelfe in the curious penning of this Treatiſe, or by the Printers neglecting, ſome faults are eſcaped, I craue as heertofore, pardon for both: knowing that I ſhall make a rude performance of a good meaning. Commending this booke to the fauorable conſideration of the friendly Readers, and my ſelfe vnto thy accuſtomed curteſie, proteſting, that meere loue and zeale vnto my countrey and countrey men profeſſors of Chirurgerie, hath mightily emboldened me, to the publiſhing of this worke, and do preſent the ſame vnder the ſhields of your protection: the which is the very ſumme, reach, and ſcope of my whole meaning, not minding to ſhew my ſelfe any way vaineglorious, or ambitious, as ſome malitious men will vncharitably deeme. And thus briefly I conclude with the waightie ſaying of Ariſtotle, that the greateſt part of thoſe things, which my ſelfe do know in this art of Chirurgerie, is the ſmalleſt portion of thoſe things, whereof I am ignorant and know not: wiſhing that it wil pleaſe almightie God, to bleſſe theſe my labours with a happie and good ſucceſſe.

Amen.

William Clowes.

OBSERVATIONS.

Now as followeth are set downe the seuerall cures, of sundry persons, which by Gods helpe haue been finished and cured.

The cure of certaine men being burned with the flame of Gun powder. Cap. 1.

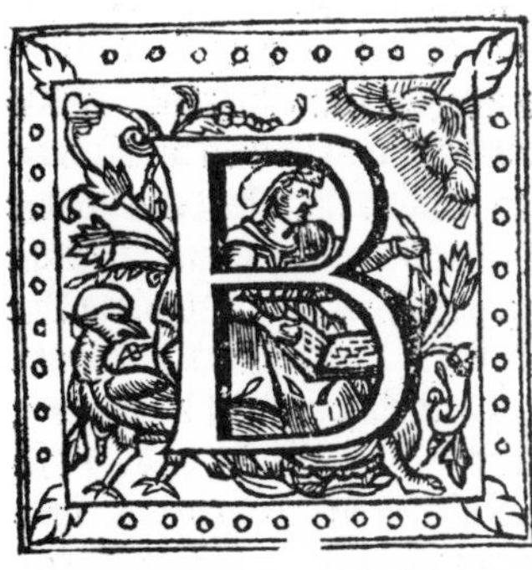

Efore I enter into this discourse, I thought it best friendly Reader, in a word or two to make cleere and plaine vnto you since the publishing of this my booke of obseruations, and also the other of *Lues Venerea*, vpon some speciall occasions, I haue againe examined and diligently perused them, & farther considering, that whilest a man liueth, any thing that is amisse may be amended: I haue therfore in some sort altered and corrected these two bookes, and so haue ioyned them both togither in one, and many things I haue left out as needlesse againe to be spoken of, also I haue enlarged these two bookes with new obseruations and approoued remedies before wanting, the which doth as it were greatly inrich the same. And for that I would be loth to obscure and hide the thing which may do good, I haue therefore heere set them out to publike view of indifferent iudges, the which worke (as I take it) is most needfull and necessarie for this present troublesome time, and may very easily be vnderstood of any Surgeon, who hath as it were but a taste or smack of any learning at all, as who so will vouchsafe at their conuenient leisure to bestowe the perusing and diligent reading thereof, I doubt not but they will thinke their labors and time well bestowed. And thus hitherto hauing very briefly declared the causes of this last publication, I will heere spend no further time, nor vse any other preambulations, but presently enter into the first beginning of this booke, with the very same matter and words in substance and meaning, as in some sort is contained in my former writings.

It

IT happened in *Anno* 1577. two Gentlemen were drying Gun powder in a braſſe pan, who (as it did appéere) had no conſideration vnto the ouer heating of the pan, but without knowledge of the danger, and care of themſelues did continually ſtir the powder with their hands: It chanced ſo, that the powder vpon a ſudden fired, wherwith they were moſt gréeuouſly burned, both hands and face, with their bodies and clothes, which cauſed them to make a moſt lamentable crying: and being heard of diuers in the ſame houſe, who perceiuing their chamber to be in a great ſmoke & ſmell of Gun powder, preſently entred in, & with all haſte that poſſible might be, caried the perſons burned into an other rome, where they forthwith did cut, rend, & teare off al their clothes frõ their bodies: otherwiſe without their helpes, no queſtion but they had béene burned to death. There dwelled néere vnto them a gentlewoman, by whom they were greatlie eaſed with a whey which ſhe made of veriuice and milke: neuertheleſſe ſhe was fearfull to procéede any further, for that ſhe neuer had ſéene the experience in the curing of ſuch great burnings with Gun powder, neither could hir ſtomack well digeſt the ſight and filthy ſauors thereof: whereupon I was preſently ſent for, and after diligent view had, I did firſt annoint the parts that were ſcorched and bliſtered oftentimes, ſpecially their hands and face, with this remedy followin , whereby the parts afflicted were preſerued from bliſtering.

Gale.

R. Salis com. ℥.ß.
Succi cæparum. ℥.iiij.
Miſce.

But where the ſkin was cleane burned off, and the parts made thereby raw and painfull, then I did apply onely this vnguent, the which I haue many times approued in diuers cures, with good ſucceſſe vnto thoſe that haue béene ſo burned with Gun powder, which medicine was neuer altered nor changed till the parts were perfectly made whole, without any further helpes.

An vnguent for burnings with Gun powder.

Clowes.

℞. Axungiæ porcinæ. lib. iiij. being firſt well waſhed in the waters of roſes and nightſhade. ana. q.s.
Olei lini lib. ij.
Olei Roſ. lib. j. ß.
Foliorum maluarum }
Violarum } ana. m. j.
Nymphex }

Plantaginis

Plantaginis
Prunellæ
Vmbilici Veneris
Cortic. sambuc. virid.
Semperuiui } ana. m. j.
Coronæ terræ, &
fol. Pomorum spinæ. } ana. m. iiij.

Infuse all these for the space of sixe daies, then boile them with a gentle fire of coles, till the herbes be parched, then straine them, and adde thereunto Ceræ albæ, q.s. Camphor. ℥.ß. dissolued in oile of Roses: and if you please in the boiling to put in of shoomakers péece grease, lib.ß. your unguent will be the better: for I haue with this unguent, as I before declared, cured many, and it is onely of mine owne inuention. But note this well, that unto their eies I applied this remedie following.

℞. Aquæ Ros. rub ℥.iiij.
Lactis muliebris. ℥.ij.
Ouorum albuminum. numero. ij.
Sacchari Candi. q.s.
Misce.

And I annointed the eie lids, and the parts néere thereunto with this excellent unguent,

℞. Olei Ros. ℥.viij.
Cerussæ lotæ in aquæ Ros. Rub. ℥.ij.
Ceræ albæ. ℥.ij.
Albuminum ouorum, numero iiij.
Camphoræ, ʒ.ij.
Misce.

In the end I finished these cures, without blemish or manifest signes of any burnings, with the often using of Oleum ouorum, & Oleum Amygdalorum dulcium, &c.

Now heere followeth certaine remedies, good for burnings with Gun powder. Cap. 2.

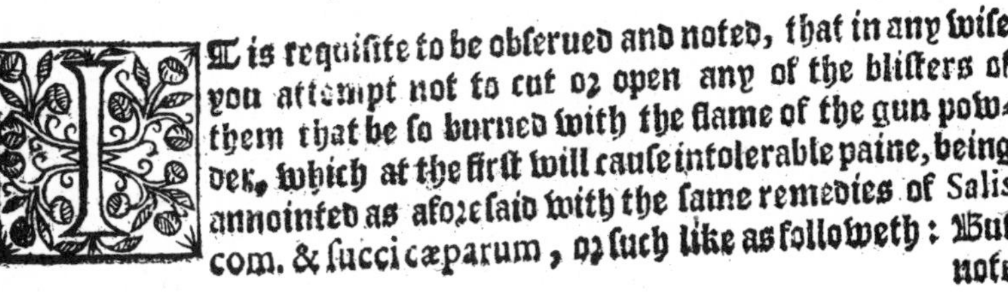

It is requisite to be obserued and noted, that in any wise you attempt not to cut or open any of the blisters of them that be so burned with the flame of the gun powder, which at the first will cause intolerable paine, being annointed as aforesaid with the same remedies of Salis com. & succi cæparum, or such like as followeth: But note

note this alwaies, that if the inflammation do so increase, that the humors vnder the blistered skin, do corrode and vlcerate the flesh, then you must in any wise cut the blisters, to giue passage vnto those painfull humors.

Mel saponis.

℞. Saponis nigr. lib.j.
Mellis com. lib. ß.
Salis com. ℥. j.
Misce.

The cure of a man greeuously burned with gun powder.

Not long since, there was a man burned with gun powder, especially on the backside of his right hand, & also his arme euen vp to his elbow, in very grieuous sort, that the skin on the backside of his hand was cleane burnt, & his arme also scorched, and blisters did presently rise in diuers places: Then with all spéede there was a Surgeon sent for, that did dwell néere vnto him, who hauing intelligence by the messenger of this mishap, he presently furnished himselfe with the aboue named Mel saponis, who at his comming to visite his patient, finding him in great extremitie of paines & burning heat, did then, with all spéede addresse himselfe for the cure of the patient, & he spred of the saide Mel saponis, vpon browne paper, and then laide it ouer all the gréeued parts, aswell vnto the rawe and tender places where the skin was cleane burned off, as also vnto the parts, which were but scorched and blistered: and thus supposing he had done well, notwithstanding the patients paines excéeded, he continued his former course of dressing from Thursday in the afternoone, vntill Saterday next following in the morning all which time & space his paines were excéeding intolerable: then at the last the Surgeon himselfe was amazed, and knew not what to do, but very early in the morning he came vnto me, and desired my counsell and helpe, and acquainted me with the cause of his comming, which was, that I should bring with me, such remedies, as would spéedily ease his patient, of the extremitie of his paines, for he confessed that it was a cure which himselfe had séene little experience of: So in regarde of his curtesie, and also being very desirous of knowledge in the Art, the which causes the rather induced me to leaue off all mine owne busines for that time, I went with him: and after my comming to the patient, perceiuing indéed his paines and gréefe to be most lamentable, as it appéred by his heauie countenance, so that I feared his graue would haue swallowed him vp: but after I had diligently viewed the maner of his burning, and did farther behold how disorderly he had béen delt with, I secretly conferred with the Surgeon, and told him he had not done well, in the applying of his Mel saponis in all places alike, for I said, although it be a medicine of ancient experience with some, and many times vsed as they

they say with great profit, chiefly to kéepe the parts that are burned and scorched from blistering, which is a most excellent thing so to do, yet it is a thing not méete to be vsed vpon the tender and rawe places: for by that meanes you do adde paines vnto paines, and heat vnto heat, or as it were fire vnto fire, like vnto him which did set his house on fire, and to quench it againe, did cast vpon it two or thrée barrels of gun powder. For which cause I haue héere set downe this note or obseruation, onely as a forewarning vnto others for committing the like fault and offence. To procéede, he was presently let bloud, and I did after take Aqua Ranarum & lactis vaccinæ ana.q.s. being mixed togither, and a little warmed, then we did wash and bathe the parts almost halfe an houre togither with cleane linnen clothes, and thus we continued thrée times a day, and thrée times a night during the time of his great extremitie of paines: after which bathing, then we did wring out the saide linnen clothes, and on the same was spred of my forenamed Vnguent, for burnings with gun powder, as it is now published in this booke. So that by this maner and order of dressing aforesaid, which was continued till the extremitie of his paines, and burning heat was well qualified, I say within the space of sixtéene daies, he was made whole by these cooling remedies, which did quench the firie heat of his great burning, onely now and then I did applie of Emp. diachalcitheos ℥.iiij. and I relented it, and then added vnto the Emp. diachalcitheos in the cooling, Vnguenti Albi Camphorati ℥. j. ß. and vsed no other meanes vnto the ende of the cure: neuerthelesse there was left behinde an vnséemely cicatrice, by reason of the ill handling at the first, which after by no meanes possible coulde be preuented or amended: then I tolde the yong man, he had serued an ill saint, which did not learne him to know any better the nature and propertie of his medicines: he answered me againe, his knowledge was iust of his masters pitch: then I spake little to him, but willed him to be more diligent in reading of good authors, and héereafter to be carefull how he applied his medicines.

Or this.

℞. Succi ceparum. ℥. ij.
Olei Lini vet. ℥.i.
Misce.

Any of these may be vsed as aforesaid, and then if you please you may safely procéede in this cure with my Vnguent, or else with any of these héere vnder written or such like.

An Vnguent for burnings with gun powder.

℞. Lithargirij auri. ℥. iiij.
Olei Ros. ℥. iij.
Olei papaueris. ℥.ij ß.

Am.Pare. Vnguenti populei.℥.iiij.
Camphor.ʒ.j.
Fiat vnguentum in mortarium plumbo secundum artem.

Or this.

Medici Florentini. ℞. Olei rosati.℥.viij.
Olei ouorum.℥.ij.
Nitri albi puluerizati.℥.ij.
Ceræ.℥.j.ss.
Corticis med. sambuci. m.j.
Misce & fiat vnguentum secundum artem.

Or this.

D.B. ℞. The pith and barke of Elders, ana.℥.ij. boile these in thrée pints of water till halfe be consumed, then straine it, and adde thereto oile of Nuts ℥.iiij. boyle these till the water be consumed, and adde thereto Ceræ, q.s.

Or this.

Iosephus Quercetanus ℞. Lard molten in the flame ℥.ij. and powre it into the iuice of Béets and Rue, the creame of Cow milke, ana. q.s. Mucilage, of the séedes of Cidonium & Dragagant, ana ℥.ss.
Misce & fiat vnguentum.

Or this.

Iacobus Weckerus. ℞. Calcis extinctæ.℥.iij.
Olei. lib.j.
Ceræ.℥.iij.

Thou shalt euery day once wash the chaulke, and let the water be taken away with a spunge, do this ten daies, then wash it in Rose water, and let it drie, and then melt your waxe and oyle, and take it from the fire, and put in the calx, made into most fine powder vnto the oile and waxe, &c. Also Calcis extinctæ made into very fine powder and mixed with Vnguentum rosarceum, is very profitable to staie the arising of the blisters.

The true maner and order of the curing a marchant of this citie of London, called M. *Thomas Gore*, which was wounded with Gun shot in the towne of Vlushing. Cap. 3.

A Fewe yéeres past a marchant of good account, in this citie of London, called M. *Thomas Gore*, being in Vlushing in Zealand, there making

making great sute vnto the prince of Orenge and the States, for the release of a ship and goods of his, and his friends, which the Vlushingers had taken at sea: in the time of that sute, he did stande at a dore where his lodging was, beholding a band of Dutch soldiers as they were marching to the wals: and as it is in townes of war the maner of some soldiers in a brauery to discharge their peeces as they passe by, so one of the soldiers that certainly knew him, and the cause of his comming to the towne, maliciously as the marchant himselfe confessed, hauing his peece charged with a bullet, suddenly shot at him, both his hands being clasped togither, and the bullet missing his bodie passed through the middle of both his hands, and fractured the bones, and also wounded him through the vpper part of his left arme, and also perced and fractured that bone in many peeces: which bullet also did rend and teare the muscles, sinewes, vaines, and arteries, by reason hereof, there followed great paines, inflations and tumors, which continued a long time, notwithstanding he was presently preserued and drest by the Surgeons of the towne of Vlushing: but he saide he receiued by them small hope or comfort of his recouery, notwithstanding I know they were excellent men: Then his friends being gentlemen and marchants of London, were by him giuen to vnderstand that he was still from day to day worse and worse, for which cause they sent for him to London, and presently vpon his arriuall, I was brought vnto this cure, and after conference had with a doctor of Physicke for his diet, purging and bleeding, I made ready forthwith this cataplasma, which appeased the paines and ceased the inflammation.

A Cataplasma.

℞. Foliorum maluarum
& violarum } ana. m. ij.
Florum chamæmeli
Fol. rof. } ana. m. j.

Boile all these in new milke till they be very soft, then stampe them in a morter and adde thereunto

Vnguenti ros.
Vnguenti populei } an. ℥. j. ß.
Vitellorum ouorum numer. ij.
Farinæ hordei ℥. ii.
Radicis Althææ, &
Seminis Psyllii } ana. ℥. ß

Somtimes I did put in of these Mucilages of ech ℥. ij. and of oyle of roses ℥. ß. with the crums of white bread steeped in new milke ℥. iij. by these meanes the parts were freed from all the paines aforesaide: which being done, to shun the like dangerous accidents, which oftentimes in such wounds are hard to be resisted, I applied round about the parts this defensiue following,

℞. Olei ros. ℥. ß.
Olei myrtini ʒ. iii.
Sanguin. draconis
Boli Armeniaci } ana. ℥. ß.
Farinæ hordei
Albuminum ouorum } ana. q. s.
Aceti ros.
Misce.

A Mundificatiue.

℞. Mel ros. ℥. ii.
Terebinthinæ ℥. iii.
Succi apii, &
Plantag. } ana. ℥. i. ß.

Boile all these togither a little, and then adde thereto,

Farinæ hord. &
Farinæ fabarum } ana. ℥. ß.
Sarcocollæ ʒ. i. ß.
Croci ʒ. ß.
Misce.

Powder that which is to be powdred, and mixe all these togither, stirring it continually till it come to perfection. Notwithstanding I had very great helpe by this mundificatiue, and the powder of Mercurii præcipitati, yet I was after constrained to vse more stronger remedies: and amongst others I found most profit in this powder following, which did not onely take away the euil flesh, but also did remoue diuers fragments and pieces of broken bones, which were not fully losed from the paniculous parts, and also hidden in the spungious flesh, neuerthelesse it worketh not without paine, therefore in such causes, if possible it may be, it is better to let nature separate the bones, than to take them away by force and violence.

This powder is good to take away spungious and corrupt flesh.

℞ Mercurij præcipitati. ʒ. iij.
Aluminis combust. in aceto Ros. ʒ. j.
Cinnabaris. ʒ. ß.
Misce.

Likewise I commonly vsed Emplastrum Diachalcitheos published in this booke, after I had taken away all the corrupt and spungious flesh, and mundified the wounds, and also remoued the lose bones, then next I vsed my Vnguentum incarnatiuum, whereunto sometimes I did mixe Aluminis combust. in Aceto Ros. which vnguent did not onely drie vp superfluous moisture, but did moreouer gently cleanse without

out any great mordication or hiting: which being performed, then I did shortly after desiccate and dry vp the said wounds with Vuguentum desiccatiuum and Emplastrum diachalcitheos, and thus I performed this worke and cured him perfectly within this citie of London.

The cure of one master Andrew Fones a marchant of London, who being in a ship at the sea was set vpon by the Vlushingers, in which fight he was very dangerously wounded with Gun shot. Cap. 4.

This Marchants ship was set vpon by certaine Vlushingers at sea, and being a long time in fight with them, and very sore oppressed by the number of men, and ships: yet they did fight it out, vntil at the last by chance he was shot into the vpper part of his brest neere vnto Os furculæ, or the channell bone, and so passed through till it came to the lower part of Os scapulæ, or the shoulder blade, where it did rest till he came to London, which was a long time: for immediately after his hurt, the ship was taken and carried into Vlushing, where he was in cure (as he said to me and many others) a long time with two of the Prince of Orenges Chirurgions, to his great cost and charges, yet it profited nothing. Then I was sent for, and after speeches had, I prepared my selfe, and forthwith made probation and found where the shot was secretly lodged: then I did without tarience, in the presence of diuers skilfull Chirurgions of London, make reasonable deepe and large incision, and there I did take out the shot, and after that there was great care had of him by his friends, for that I did giue them to vnderstand that the wound was not without danger. Then they ioined with me one of hir Maiesties Phisitions, who directed him to take Arcæus Apozema, which certainly did worke most excellently wel, the proofe thereof I neuer had seene vntill that time, but many times since I haue vsed it, and I haue found thereof a treasure for the curing of wounds in the brest, which composition I will here set downe for the worthinesse thereof, as it was ministred to him. But first after I had taken out the shot, I preserued the wound with this digestiue, the which I vsed vpon tents and pledgets.

℞ Terebinthinæ lotæ in aqua vitæ ℥.iiij.
Vitellorum ouorum.num.ij. A digestiue: Clowes.
Olei.Ros.℥.ß.

Mercurii

Mercurii præcipitat.biscalcinati.ʒ.j.
Croci.℈.j.
Misce.

And after the wound was herewith preserued, then I annointed the parts greeued round about with warme oile of Roses, and ouer all a plaister of Diachalcitheos dissolued in oile of Roses, q.s. and at euery dressing I applied hot steuphs of white wine and aqua vitæ, q.s. Then I defended the wound from accidents with this defensiue,

A defensiue.

℞ Pul.Ros.rub.& Myrtillorum } ana.ʒ.j.
Boli Armeniaci Terræ sigelatæ } ana.ʒ.vj.
Succorum plantaginis & Solani. } ana.℥.j.
Olei Ros.omphac. & Myrtillorum } ℥.ii.ß.
Aceti Ros.℥.j.
Ceræ.℥.ij.
Misce.

In which time and space of the vse of these outward remedies, I did giue him to drinke of this Apozema, often times q.s.

Apozema Arcæi.

℞ Hordei mundati contusi Passularum mundatarum, contusarum } ana.p.iiij.
Radicum buglossæ contusarum m.iij.
Glycyrrhizæ rasæ modice contusæ ℥.j.ß.
Cardui benedicti m.ij.
Seminum communium ℥.ii.
Iuiubas numero xx.
Prunorum numero xv.
Radicum Petroselini contus.m.i.

All which being boiled in xiiii.pounde of raine water, to the consumption of the third part, let them be strongly strained, whereunto shall be added,

Penidiorum ℥.iii.
Sirupi rosat. Sirupi de duabus radicibus sine aceto } ana.℥.iii.
Sacchari albi lib.ß.
Cinnamomi pulucrizati ʒ.i ß.
Fiat Apozema.

And likewise for clensing and mundifying of the said wound, I vsed this mundificatiue following, & also many times besides Vnguentum basilicon

basilicon mixed with Mercurie præcipitat.&c.

℞ Terebinthinæ Venet.lotæ in aqua fumaria ℥.iiii.
Vitellorum ouorum numero ii.
Mellis Rof. } ana.℥.ii.
Sir. de fumaria }
Farinæ Orobi. ℥.iii.
Thuris }
Masticis } ana.℥.ß.
Aloes hæpaticæ }
Radicis Peucedani.ʒ.i.
Misce.

Mundificatiuum Petri Andreæ.

Also I iniected inwardly with a syring this excellent lotion, which did wonderfully well mundifie and clense the brest.

℞. Hordei mundati } ana.℥.ii.
Lentium }
Caudæ equinæ.m.i.
Rof.Rub.m.ß.

Iniectio mundificatiua.

Boile them in equall parts of common and Plantaine water cum modico succi mali punaci, vnto the consumption of the third part, putting thereto when it is strained,

Sacchari rub.℥.ii.
Sirup.ex infusione rof.℥.iii.
Croci ℈.ß.

After the parts were perfectly mundified, then I perfected the cure with these remedies héere vnder prescribed.

℞. Aqua hordei lib.ß.
Sirup.Rof.℥.i.
Penidiorum ℥.ii.
Liqueritiæ ʒ.ii.
Myrrhæ ℥.ß.
Misce.

Iniectio incarnatiua & mundificatiua.

Moreouer, with the afore rehearsed iniections I vsed this vnguent, which is very necessarie for such wounds made with Gun shot: and I haue approued it in many other cures, as it was prescribed in the former copie, and as it is now in this booke corrected and published.

℞. Succi de Peto lib.vi.
Adipis ouini lib.ii.
Olei com.lib.ii.
Terebinthinæ Venetiæ ℥.xii.
Resinæ Pini lib.i.
Masticis ℥.ii.

Vnguentum de Peto & Nicotiana.

Clowes.

Colophoniæ

Colophoniæ lib.ii.
Ceræ lib.i.
Vini albi lib.i.
Misce & fiat vnguentum secundum artem.

Let not the Succi de Peto be put in, before all the rest be well relented togither, and then strained into a cleane pan, and being molten, put in the iuices to the rest, and boile it till the iuices be all consumed: then straine it againe, and reserue it to your vse. With these remedies before rehearsed, I did perfectly make him whole, & I cicatrized vp the wound with Vnguentum desiccatiuum rub. and so he remained perfectly cured twelue yéeres, vntill his dying day, which was in *Anno* 1595. within the citie of London, &c.

The cure of a certaine soldier that was wounded with Gun shot in the Low countries: he was shot in at the bottom of his belly on the left side, and the bullet passed through, and rested in the right buttock neere vnto Anus, where it lay secretly hid, and could not be found for the space of three yeeres, in which time it became a Fistula of a hard curation. Cap. 5.

In the yéere of our Lord 1573. I was sent for, vnto my singular good friend Master Richard Yoong, one of hir Maiesties Iustices of peace for Middlesex, who did earnestly request me, that I would for his sake, cure and heale, if it were possible, the aforesaid soldier, called M. Giles, for that he was knowen to be a very valiant man, which cure to performe, séemed to me very hard and difficult, for that he had béen for the space of thrée yéeres, with diuers very good Surgeons, both beyond the seas as also in England, and yet his griefe did still reuerse, and breake out againe: the reason I perceiued was, for that the place, where the bullet lay, could neither by probation, nor coniecture be certainly knowen, and that was the chiefest cause I suppose, why they failed in this cure: so at this Gentlemans request, I did take him in cure, and after due consideration and search made, with probes of Lead, and waxe candles, and long and small flexible tents, that were apt to yéeld to euery crooked turning, yet by no meanes I could come to the knowledge or vnderstanding where the bullet had conuaied and hid it selfe, neither could the patient himselfe giue me any certaine direction thereof:

thereof: then first of all I enlarged the mouth or orifice of the fistula, with a tent made of a spunge, and for that the callous hollownes did penetrate déepe, and (as I haue said) being vncertaine of the bottome, which was in the part where the bullet lay: Therefore I ordained a long and small stiffe tent made of fine lint without any grosse thréeds in it, and so with the white of an egge well beaten, I framed my tent in length and bignes, according to the greatnes and smalnes of the griefe: which being thus prepared according to art, then I did annoint euery tent slightly ouer, with Vnguentum Rosarum, onely to haue the powders cleaue fast, and take better hold on the tents, wherby it might be so conueied in, to remoue and destroy the callous hardnes, which was inuironed about the circuits or compasse of the hollownes of the fistula, and the first powder that I vsed for this purpose, was the powder which I haue published in the third Chapter of this booke, pag.8. After I had reasonably well enlarged the fistula with the foresaid powder, which I vsed twise a wéeke: and allwaies I remoued the scars with vnguentum rosarum, and laid vpon the same most commonly Emplastrum Diachalcitheos dissolued with oile of roses, and Rose vineger, and the whites of egs, being mixed well togither, and so I applied it: and although I had herewith partly taken away the callous matter, yet I found not that profit and commoditie as heretofore I had done, in the curing of diuers other. Then hauing full hope of better successe with this strong powder next following, the which I applied after the same maner and order as the other aforesaid.

The strong powder.

℞ Vitrioli albi combust. ℥.i.
Aluminis vsti ℥.ß.
Mercurii. sublimat. ℈.i.
Bolei Armeniaci orient. q.s.
Misce.

With this powder I did wholy destroy the callous matter, so far as it was possible to conuey in my tents. Then I supposed that I had made sufficient proofe to haue found where the bullet rested, but do what I could by searching, either whẽ he stood vpright, or stowped downwards, or as he stood when he was shot, the which he did so néere as he could direct me: all this profited nothing, till at the last I did consider that such Fistulas that hath mo crékes or turnings than one, could hardly be cured by tents. Wherefore I followed the counsell of Tagaltius, who saith in the cure of Fistulas, where medicine by tents cannot be brought, or conueied into the bottom as the cause doth require: then to vse iniections and liquors méet for the purpose, to be cast in with a spring, is (saith he) greatly auailable, as I very well did proue by this cure: for I prepared this water following, the which I did cast in with a syring that had a long pipe and a large barrell: the said water is called aquæ fallopii.

Aquæ Fallopij.

℞ Aquæ plantaginis
& ros. } ana.lib.i.
Aluminis roch.
Argenti sublimati } ana.ʒ.ii.

Put al these togither in a double glasse, and boile it in Balneo mariæ, to the consumption of the fourth part. After I had cast in of this water, presently I stopped the mouth or orifice of the Fistula, to this end and purpose that thereby the skin might also become the more thin, by reason of the long lying in of the iniection, and store of matter which was gathered within the cauity or bottom of the Fistula. And (as I said) caused him forthwith to lie downe vpon his right buttock, according as the passage directed me, onely that the water should not returne back againe till it had wrought his effect, for within xiiij. houres after he did greatly complaine of extreme paine in his right buttocke neere vnto Anus, and there I did perceiue it to be greatly tumified and swolne, then I applied on the outside of his buttocke where he complained a Cataplasma, which is singular good in such causes. The composition is as followeth,

Anodynum Cataplasma.

Clowes.

℞ Foliorum maluarum
Hyoscyami albi } ana. m.i.ß.
Florum chamæmeli
& Ros. } ana.m.i.

Boile these in new milke, then ad thereto.

Medullæ panis q.s.
Farinæ hordei ℥.ii.
Sem.lini ℥.iii.
Oleorum ros.
& Violarum } ana. ℥.i.ß.
Vitellorum ouor. numero iii.
Croci ℈.i.
Misce.

Thus I let him remaine till the next day following in the morning, for then I had good hope that the water had found the passage and place where the bullet had seated it selfe, then I called others in presence when I made incision vpon the right buttock neere vnto Anus, where the swelling shewed it selfe. There I made incision, and did take out the shot, and for that time to mitigate the paine, I iniected new milke and Suger with a little oile of Roses, and vpon pledgets I applied Vnguentum

tum rosarum, to remooue the eschars which were made by the foresaide water, and I staied the bleeding which followed after the incision with *Galens* powder: and so he rested reasonable quiet all that day and the next night: then at the second dressing I ordained this vnguent, the which I vsed till the paines and inflammation were ceased, and the said vnguent is made of Axungiæ porcinæ & oculi populei, q.s. wherewith I mixed a small quantitie of Mercurij præcipitati, then after I did mundifie it with this mundificatiue.

Vnguentum Populeon simplex.

℞. Gum. ammoniaci ℥.ii.
Galbani ℥.i. ß.
Aloes }
Sarcoc. } ana. ℥.i.
Terebinthinæ ℥.iiii.
Resinæ pini ℥.ß.
Olei ros. ℥.iii.
Olei mastic. ℥.iiii.
Mellis ros. ℥.i.
Succorum plantaginis }
Apii }
Card. bened. } ana. ℥.ß.
Viridis æris ʒ.iii.

Vnguentum mundificatiuum.

Dissolue your Gums in white wine, and make an vnguent according to art. After that the parts were well mundified, then I did iniect into the griefe twise a day this iniection, which doth both incarnate and conglutinate.

℞ Aquæ hordei lib. i.
Mel ros. ℥.iii.
Sarcocol. ʒ.ii.
Olibani & }
Myrrhæ } ana. ʒ.i.
Vini maluatici ℥.vi.

The iniection Tagaltius.

Thus in a short time time I finished this cure, with this iniection and with my vnguent Nicotion or De peto and the plaister of Diachalcitheos, &c.

A very hard and dangerous cure which happened to a common soldier called *John Searle*, by a shot with a Musket bullet, through the ioint of his shoulder on his right arme, which fractured a great part of the said ioint into many peeces. Cap. 6.

A Few yeeres past, there was sent vnto me by M. *Marre* a gentleman attending vpō general *Norrice*, who not long before I cured of a wound in his hand, I say he sent vnto me by his man a certaine soldier called *Iohn Searle*, being in the flower of his age (about some six and twentie yeeres) and of a reasonable good constitution of body, who was shot through the ioint of his right shoulder with a musket bullet, so that a great part of the bones of the said ioint were battered and broken into many peeces, with the force of the bullet: It was said, he receiued this wound at the siege of Graue, he seruing then vnder the conducting and leading of Generall *Norrice*, being there cheefe commander of the English regiment, at which time the Generall himselfe was wounded on the brest with a pike, and escaped his life most dangerously, he was then also thrust into the mouth and throte with a pike, so that two of his foremost teeth were fractured & broken in peeces with the force of the pike, whom I cured in the Low Countries. (As I haue before said) at the earnest request of M. *Marre* I diligently viewed and searched the aboue named soldier his greefe, which for want of orderly preseruing and dressing, and good looking vnto: and moreouer lacke of abilitie to pay for the curing of so great & dangerous a greefe, was like to haue perished: by reason therof his wound was in time ouergrown with corrupt and spungious flesh: the humors also were continually fleeting, corrupt, and of a stinking sauor, the whole ioint was maruellously swolne, and sore oppressed with very great paine: by reason of the humors that were gathered about the ioint, being vehemently heated, and full of rancor and malice, which proceeded partly of those causes afore declared, and also of the causes after following: moreouer, his arme from the shoulder, and so downe vnto his hande was vnmeasurably swolne, the skin indurate and hard, so that he had smal feeling of that arme, but with a dull sense: and also his arme was vnweldy and heauy: the orifices of the said wound were very small, and almost closed vp togither. After I perceiued all these pernitious signes and accidents, wherewith the

whole

whole member was assailed, and which to my iudgement threatened great dangere, whereby I doubted it would proue but a sorrowful cure, yet for that he was a man of a valiant and stout courage, and farther calling to minde the wise sayings of *Iosephus Quercetanus*, a man as it may appéere, liuing in the light of all good learning, he declareth in the second chapter of his booke of curing Gun shot: That he would not haue the wounded patient forsaken as a dead man, although the wound séeme dangerous and mortall, but with all diligence to apply méete and conuenient medicines, For saith he, many times nature being hol- A historie.
" pen by Art, worketh myracles, whereby emperickes to the great infa-
" my of Physicke oftentimes purchase fame, for being bold vpon the
" strength of nature, they take in hand desperate cures, forsaken as dead
" men by the Physitions, and get thereby to themselues great credite, & to
" the Physitions no lesse shame, as by heare-say about two yéeres past it
" happned to a noble prouinciall named *Vnissius*, who being in the kings ar-
" mie against *Rupella*, was by a shot pearced through, & forsaken of the phy-
" sitions, who iudged the substance of his liuer to be perished, and yet was
" cured by some of his noble fréends with medicines of no great price:
" The which rare euent, may be a notable example of the strange effects
" of nature, which oftentimes deceiueth the iudgement of most learned
" Physitions, whom I would wish neuer to be destitute of singular reme-
" dies against desperate and hainous gréefes, &c.

Héereby may be perceiued that famous men of all former ages, vntill this day reproue all those Physitions and Surgeons in like sort, which at any time refuse to helpe and succor their wounded patients, though the wound séeme deadly and dangerous: for if he happen to die for want of all helpe, we may iustly saith *Guido*, be accounted and taken for most wicked and vncharitable persons: And so I will héere leaue to speake any farther of this matter, for that my onely meaning is héere to instruct yoong practizers, and not otherwise to discourse, as I haue before said, I hauing a carefull foresight, and being very desirous to do all the good I could vnto this poore man, and also loth to prolong and abuse the time, as that vilde slander goeth vpon Surgeons generally, but chiefly of the Surgeons of London vndeserued, amongst whom I know there are many which are worthy to be recorded in the number of most excellent famous men: whereof I could speake more largely, but that this place serueth not to declare by-matters, and therefore to procéede vnto the end. Therefore with all diligence I did make probation, and searched the said wound, which done, I did forthwith fortifie, strengthen and defend the weake parts, by applying about the ioint repelling medicines, to the intent to staie the streame, and intercept the

flux

flux of humors that was stirred vp, partly by often searching, and also by sharpe and biting medicines as followeth, which of very necessitie must needes be done, then I indeuored my selfe to enlarge the orifices of the said wound, and to subdue the corrupt and spungeous flesh, which was performed with great care and diligence: first I made a long tent, the which I armed with the common caustick, made vnguent wise, and so I conueied it into the farthest part of the wound, so far as it was possible, at that present time to go. The strange euent of the said ruptury or caustick is not onely in this cure, but in many others greatly to be esteemed: thus after the orifices of the said wound were sufficiently enlarged for the time present, then to appease the paines and heat that were greatly increased by the often vsing againe and againe of sharpe and biting medicines, which was done to this end and purpose, to discouer the things infixed which a long time had been hidden within the said ioint, as followeth, first to remoue the eschars aforesaid, and to digest the humors, I applied vpon tents and dossels, Vnguentum populeon simplex sometimes mixed with Mercurij precipitati q. s. next thereunto I applied a plaister of Diachalcitheos, dissolued with oile of Roses, and the iuice of Housleeke, and Plantaine, ana. q.s. and so to couer ouer all the ioint of the arme downe to the hand: this Cataplasma whose cooling facultie exceedeth in restraining the inflammation, and also to mittigate the paine.

℞. Micæ panis infusæ in lacte vaccino lib.i.ß.

Boile it a little, then adde thereto

A cataplasma

Olei viol.
Olei Ros. } ana ℥.iii.
Vitellor.ouor.numero iiii.
Puluer.rosar.rub.
Flor.Chamamell.&
Melilot. } ana.℥.ii.
Far.fabar.&
Hordei } ana.℥.j.

Mingle all these togither, and make a Cataplasma according to art. Thus as I haue said, I continued from time to time, till the extreme paines were somwhat asswaged, and the weake member a little strengthened, which by long infirmitie and ill looking vnto, was greatly feebled, for these causes I did many times forbeare the often vsing of forcible and strong medicines, knowing indeede that the best way of curing, is if it be possible, to cure quickly and without paine, or as little as may be. But after his paines and swelling were somewhat taken away, partly by the foresaid Cataplasma, and partly by a plaister of Demineo,

made

made with the oiles of neates tœte and linesœde, of equall portions, &c. But it is furthermore to be noted, that first of all he was purged by the counsell of a physition, and then next I did foment all the parts round about his ioint, and so likewise downe his arme to his hand with a fomentation, which I made of malusey, vineger, and oile of roses ana.q.s. Whereby the pores of the skin, were the better opened, that the humors might the easilier breath forth, and be resolued: which done, I went about the more boldly to subdue and take away the superfluous and spungious flesh, whereby the corruption being inclosed, had the frœer passage. The which was done sometimes with Mercurij præcipitati alone, and sometimes I mixed with Mercurij præcipitati Vitriolium, of ech equall portions, or rather lesse of the Vitriall than of the Præcipitat. and sometimes I vsed Vitriolium album, & Bole Armoniacum made in very fine powder, as it is described in the viij. Chapter of this bœke, for the cure of a fistula: also I did vse at sundrie times Vnguentum Ægyptiacum after *Auicen*, whose properties excœde in subduing spungious flesh, and in scaling corrupt bones: in like maner I vsed many times the trochies of Deminio after *Vigo*: but in conclusion, the chiefest thing that finished and perfected this cure, was a tent made onely of the powder of Vitriall and Bole, as it is described in the Chapter aboue said, the which I made in length and greatnes vnto the concauitie of the grœued part, by meanes hereof, as it were by a miraculous operation, happily there was stirred vp aboue Os furculæ, and a little below the orifice of the wound in the corrupt ioint a rotten abscisse, wherin was compact a masse of most horrible filthie stinking matter with, certaine pœces of foule blacke & rotten bones, & pœces of the bullet of Lead, with a pœce of iron of his armour: then after I had thus wholy displaced and taken away all these annoiances, which was done, as I haue afore said, with the often visiting of the wound with eating and consuming medicines, as he was able to beare and endure it, by meanes hereof he was deliuered from all perils whatsoeuer, which a long time lay pend and lurking within the said ioint, they conspiring much hurt and danger not onely vnto the weake member, but also vnto the whole state of his bodie. And here I end this briefe note or obseruation, without farther repetition, onely I say after the wound was deliuered from all perils whatsoeuer, then the rest of the cure was accomplished according to the generall method of other cōmon wounds, as with mundificatiues, incarnatiues, and consolidatiues, &c. published in this bœke in diuers places: thus by carefull handling, and the benefit of nature he was cured of this dangerous wound, yet he remaineth still lame of that arme, and will be so all the daies of his life.

The cure of one *Henry Rodes,* one of the waiters at the Cuſtome houſe, he being vpon the riuer of Thames a skirmiſhing with his peece, and by reaſon the peece had certaine flawes in it, did breake into many peeces, and made a great wound vpon his chin, and carried away a good part of the Manduble and the teeth withall: moreouer, it did rend his hand greatly: all which I cured without maine or deformitie.

Cap. 7.

After I had ſearched the wound of his hand and face, then I preſerued thoſe wounds with oile of Hypericon warmed, and vpon the ſame to reſtraine the bleeding I applied this reſtrictiue,

A Reſtrictiue. Bolognini.

℞. Boli Armeniaci ℥.i.ß.
Sanguinis draconis } ana.ʒ.i.
Terræ ſigillatæ }
Thuris gummoſi ʒ.ii.
Pilorum leporis ℈.ß.
Ouorum Albuminum q.s.
Miſce.

And the wounds of the hand were defended from dangerous accidents, which commonly follow ſuch wounds, and will admit no cure till they be remoued by good induſtrie and diligence, which was performed with that defenſiue, which is publiſhed in Cap. 4. pag. 10.

Then with decent bolſtering and rowling I preſerued his hand for the firſt dreſſing, laying it orderly vpon a palmeſtrie of wood, well wrapped with fine towe, and then I did binde it very eaſily, ſo that his hand might ſafely lie on it without ſtirring, or remouing any way, then after the wound of his lip was alſo ſtitched. I vſed vnto the wound of the outward part, the oile of Hypericon well warmed, which I applied to with pledgets of fine lint dipped in the ſame oile, and vpon the ſaide pledgets I laid alſo the aboue named reſtrictiue plaiſter wiſe, and often dreſſed the wound in the inſide of his mouth, with Sirup. roſ. & mel. roſ. and alſo very often with this Gargariſme following,

℞ Aquæ hordei lib.i.
Succi granatorum ℥.ii.
Mellis roſ. ℥.ii.
Diamoron ℥.i.

Aquæ

Aquæ rof.& }
Plantaginis } ana. ℥.iiii.
Aluminis roch. ℥.ß.
Misce.

And thus with bolstering the wound of his chin and conuenient rowling, it rested till the second day. Then at the next preseruation I ordained steuphs of white wine and Aqua vitæ, ana.q.s. and also Vnguentum de peto or Nicotion, which I vsed continually with the oile of Hypecicon warmed, & the plaister of Diachalcitheos, and annointing the parts about with oile of Roses, and so this wound of his chin was in a short time perfectly cured: in like maner I prepared at the first for the curing of his hand also steuphs of white wine with Aqua vitæ: and I ordained likewise this digestiue, wherwith I continued vntill these wounds did yéeld perfect matter: in which time no accident followed that did any way hinder the ordinarie course of curing.

℞ Terebinthinæ lotæ in aqua vitæ ℥.ii. — A digestiue.
Vitellorum ouorum numero ii.
Croci ℈.ß.
Olei rof.℥.ß.
Farinæ hord.q.s.
Misce.

A conuenient digestiue in such wounds is necessary bicause of the alteration of the aire, and for brusing and renting of the parts so disseuered: howbeit, digestiues may not be vsed ouer long, for then they will certainly too much putrifie the parts. Moreouer, I vsed in the time of application of this digestiue, Oleum lumbricorum, & Oleum hypericonis, of each equall portions, and twise a day I dipped the pledgets of the digestiue in those foresaid oiles, & I annointed the part round about the wound with warme oile of Roses, and a plaister of Diachalcitheos dissolued in oile of Roses, with vineger & the white of an egge being wel incorporated togither, and so I continued with bolstering and rowling till the wound was well digested. Then I did mundifie these woundes of his hand with this mundificatiue, which maister *Rassius*, one of the French kings Surgeons did giue vnto me, and it is singular good in such wounds, as I haue many times approoued.

℞ Pul.aloes }
Mirrhæ & } ana.ʒ.iii. — A mundificatiue. Frances Rassius.
Gentianæ }
Pul.vtriusque Aristolochię }
& Centaurii minoris } ana.ʒ.ii.
Pul.Ireos Florent. ℥.ß.

Accipiantur omnia cum sir.
Rof.siccar.& absynthii } ana, q.s.
Addendo aquæ vitæ ℥.i.
& fiat linamentum.

After the wound was well mondified, then I prosecuted vnto the end of the cure with mine incarnatiue, and sometimes I mixed with it Alumen combust. and after brought it vnto a perfect cicatrize with vnguentum deminio héere following, and thus he was perfectly cured, both of the one, and the other wounds aforesaid.

A very good vnguent called vnguentum deminio.

R Minij leuissime triti ℥.ij.
Olei rosati
Olei mirtini } ana. ℥.ij.
Coquantur lento igne cum ceræ albæ ℥.ß.
Misce, & fiat vnguentum secundum artem.

An obseruation of the curing of Henry Battey Cheesmonger wounded in the corner of his eie, with the screw or breech of a Dag.

Now héere I will drawe to the end and full finishing of this cure, the which I performed within this city of London: at the same very instant time, I cured one *Henry Battey*, a Chéesemonger, dwelling at Broken Warfe, which by ouercharging of his Dag, it did breake into many péeces, and the bréech or screw of the Dag did mount or flie vp into the corner of his eie, and fractured the bone, and so passed vp into his head, and the wound presentlie was shut vp and closed togither: insomuch that those surgeons which thē had him in cure before I was called, supposed the wound to be very small & of no account, and indéed went about to heale it vp: but still he did grow weaker and weaker, insomuch the Bell towled for him: then I was sent for, and to be short, forthwith I enlarged the wound by incision, and I tooke out the screw of the Dag out of his head, and the péeces of the fractured bones, which were caried in with the said screw: to conclude, in a very short time after I cured him within this citie of London, and he liueth vnto this day.

The cure of a soldier being wounded with a poisoned arrow vpon the coast of Brasile, which wound after became a Fistula, very hard and difficult to be cured. Cap.8.

It is many times séen by experience frienly Reader, that of wounds receiued in the wars, do grow a number of such intricate Fistulas of very hard curation, and many of them are so inuironed with such a tough hard callous substance, with corruption of the bones in diuers parts of the body, that they are giuen ouer and forsaken of very

good

good Surgeons, as past all helpe or hope of any recouerie: and now here I giue you to vnderstand that in the yéere 1591. the xii. of Ianuary, there was sent vnto me from Captaine *Fleming*, a certaine soldier which had a fistulas vlcer in his thigh, with the hurt and corruption of the bone, being fiue inches aboue the ioint of his knée on his right leg, but before I speake any further of this matter, or of the maner of his curing, I will first a little discourse of the originall beginning, and chiefe cause of the saide fistula, and of the great danger he with others escaped in the time of their voyage. You shall here note, that after I had reasoned with this patient, he reported vnto me that the first beginning and cause of this fistula in his thigh, was by a wound with an arrow, made of a smal cane or réed, hauing a flint head, very curiously fastened on, and feathered with two long parrots feathers, or some such like, which the wilde sauage people of Brasile, and the countries néere thereunto adioining, do often poison with the iuice of an herbe, and vseth them as their chéefest weapons of defence, as I haue before declared. This soldier being vpon the coast of Brasile in a man of war, a ship of the west countrey, who a long time had béen sailing vpon the seas, and ouerdriuen with very foule weather, and hauing extreme néede of fresh water and victuals, insomuch that they were constrained vpon great occasion, to send their bote ashore early in the morning, and manned their bote with certaine shot, and other weapons of war: they being come ashore, there were certaine appointed of their company to staie behinde with the bote to fill water, and the rest trauelled vp into the countrey to sée what they could méete with to supply their wants: it was said they had not iournied very far, but they had discouered a certaine number of sauage wilde naked people, of whom at the first they made no reckoning or account of at all, bicause they séemed to be afraid, and so did flie away, and now and then staying, onely (as it was farther reported) they did it but to allure and draw forward on our men néerer vnto the rest of their force and strength, which lay in ambush for them, who nothing suspecting that they did it to betraie our men, till at the last (as he said) they had espied the rest of their company, which were gathered togither in a troupe in a very short space: then our men being some fortie fiue made a stande: neuerthelesse, those wilde people being aboue two or thrée hundred, very fiercely with a certaine noise or crie, charged our men with their arrowes and darts, &c. But our men withstood them at the first very manfully, and did hurt and kill many of them with their shot and other weapons: their number still increased with fresh wilde people, so that thereby our men perceiuing their number to be too great for them any longer to incounter withall, which fight was continued a long

long time, at the last our men were constrained to retire, in which retrait some were slaine, some hurt, and some taken, and could neuer be heard of againe: thus with much adoo the rest escaped and recouered their bote, which happily rescued our men, by reason the saide bote had certaine small péeces of ordinance in the head of it, which often they shot off, and so constrained those wilde people to retire back again, or else our men had vtterly béen ouerthrowne, so they went aboord their ship with their fresh water, and presently they called for the surgeon of their ship to dresse their hurt men, for that some of them that were sore wounded with arrowes, and darts, were in very great paines and burning heat, and shortly after, a maruellous inclination to vomiting, and much vaine and idle talke. Moreouer, the colour of their skin about their wounds was somwhat swartish, which accident appéered not vntil the second day after they receiued their hurts, but vpon none so much as vpon this soldier, which after had the fistula in his thigh: so in the end some were cured, some died shortly after, and some by no meanes possible could be healed during all the time they were at sea, neither could their wounds be brought to any good digested matter, the reason as I gathered was, that they were touched with the scuruie. To procéed, the surgeon of their ship, being as they said a man of a fine skil, and one that had great experience for the curing of such poisoned wounds, by reason he had trauelled diuers times into those countries, and did know very well that their maner was to poison their arrowes, and therefore he did at the very first with great care, make large and déepe incision, for that the breach that was made with the arrow was but little in compasse, though déepe vnto the bone: and for that cause after incision was made, he did presently fill the wound with hot Ægyptiacum, and vpon it a plaister of fine Triackle, and so drest him vp very orderly as it was reported. As for the rest that were wounded, I meane not héere to speake any further of them at all: also to defend the hart and other parts inwardly from venome and poison, he gaue this soldier amongst the rest, to eat a certaine preseruatiue, but what that was, I could not gather by his spéech. But to omit here to speake farther of preseruatiues inwardly, I haue thought it very expedient to make knowne vnto the friendly Reader, that at what time soeuer yée shall happen vpon the like cures of poisoned wounds, that you do not forget first to scarifie the edges of the wound, according as it is noted in the 12. Chapter following, to the intent to make the wound bléede the better, for that much poison is euacuated with the blood, and you must be very mindfull in all your incisions vnto the vaines and arteries, whereby may insue too immoderate profusion of blood. Then after you haue made scarification, yée shall presently set on a strong cupping glasse, the better to draw out the venome and poison, and then in the steed of the hot *Ægyptiacum*, which no doubt is very good, I thinke it likewise profitable to make triall of this excellent remedie heere following, which although I haue neuer experienced my selfe, nor sawe it practised by others, yet it is commended to me by men of skill, and it standeth with great reason, and is already published by *Iohanes Franciscus Rota*. in his booke De tormentorum Vulneribus.

An excellent remedie against poisoned wounds. Iohannes Franciscus Rota.

℞ Lixinii saponarii lib.ß.
Succi solani cum sem. ℥.ii.
Theriacæ ℥.ß.

Mixe all these togither, and put them in an earthen pot, or vessel well glased, and let it macerate in the sun by the space of twentie daies, then when you will vse of this medicine dip your pledgets, runlets or tents therein, and fill the wound accordingly, and this do till the third day. To procéede, it is furthermore to be remembred, that after this soldier and the rest of his company departed from the coast of Brasile, and so for England, they were a long time after vpon the seas, and indured maruellous stormes and tempests, and much adoo they had to bring home their ship, and recouer the coast of England, in which time many of their men fell sicke of the scuruie, so that by reason thereof, and the causes afore spoken, that of fower score and twelue men, they had not eight and twentie strong and able persons to bring home the ship: But after this soldier came a shore, and landed in the west Countrey, being sicke of the scuruie, and very ill troubled with his wounde, immediately he was taken in cure, and continued so sixtéene wéekes, in all which time and space he was nothing the better of his wound: onely he was cured of the scuruie: of which disease or infection, I meane bréefly to speake in the 12. Chapter of this booke: and now to say in a word for the cure, of this fistula, yée shall note, after he had shewed it vnto me, I founde there a very straight and narrow orifice, with foule, hard and callous lips: the humors that flowed were sanious and glutinous, with corruption of the bone of his thigh, as I haue before declared at large. So when I had thus viewed it, he desired me to tell him plainly, if he were curable or not, I answered him againe, that I was out of all doubt thereof, if he would be content to indure some paines: Alas good sir (said he) I do full well know, if painfull, strong, and forcible remedies would haue cured me, I should not now haue néeded to craue your friendship at this time, for I suppose I haue indured as many biting corsiue medicines as had béene able to haue killed a horse: Although said I you haue indured neuer so great paines, yet they must be strong and forcible medicines

dicines that must cure you, or else God knowes when you can be made whole: But to answer such obiections: I say, *Calmetius*, a singular man for his knowledge in Physicke and Chirurgery, saith these words: ,, When it seemeth expedient to make incision in a fistula, and to cut away ,, callous matter, or otherwise to vse hot irons, or strong powders and ,, caustícke medicines, and the patient is disobedient or vnwilling, and ,, will not indure and abide it, then the best way is to auoid the cure, and ,, not to make or meddle with it. So at the last he was perswaded, and very willingly was contented to indure whatsoeuer I thought meete & conuenient, for the speedy restoring him againe to his former health, &c. Then first of all I defended the greeued part, by applying rounde about his thigh that defensiue published in the third Chapter of this booke: which done, I made a tent in length and bignes of the said fistula, and I annointed it ouer with Vnguentum populeon simp. and so rowled it in, cum puluere siue pare, as it is published in this booke. And vpon the same this plaister which is commended by *Paracelsus*, to be singular good for to draw out bullets, arrow heads, and broken splinters of weapons. ℞. Wax. lib. j. of Colophone, and Shoomakers pitch ana. ℥.iii. dissolue them togither, and then adde thereunto of Gum. Amoniacke, ℥.ij. Bdellium ℥.j. of Lapis Magnetis in fine powder ℥.v. of yellow Amber ℥.iij. mixe all togither with oile of egs, and make it vp according to art, and so reserue it to your vse. I say the aforesaid powder wrought with some sharpnes and biting, then to remoue the eschars, which were made by the said powder, I drest him twise a day with Vnguentum populeium simp. till the eschar was remoued: so that within fower or fiue times vsing of this powder, I might easily feele with my probe the bone ragged, and somwhat lose, neuertheles there were diuers turnings, and much callous matter towards the bottome, the which I could by no meanes subdue, till I made a tent onely of Vitrioli albi crudi ʒ.ij. Bole Armeniaci ʒ.ß. Misce. After this maner, I did take a quantitie of this powder, and moistened it with fasting spittle, and then I wrought it to the forme of a paste, and thereof I made a tent the full length and compasse of the fistula, and so I let it rest till it was well hardened and dried, and then I conuaied it into the bottome of the fistula, where it wrought with some force, for by the firie facultie thereof, the callous matter was wholy destroied, and the continuall flowing of those humors were thereby staied, yet the bone was not ready to come away: for that cause twise a weeke I vsed vpon tents of the foresaid powder, siue pare, which at the last it brought out the scale of the bone, being somewhat blacke and ragged. And then after by the onely application of Emplastrum Stiaticum Paracelsi, laid vpon the orifice of the fistula, nature wrought

Some vse to make the like tent, but they frame it as aforesaid with the vnguent of Populeon.

wrought the rest of the cure, and so within a reasonable time after, he was perfectly healed. But note this one accedent followed by reason of the extremity of the working of the said tent made of the powder, which I precisely obserued: for the same night he fell into cramps and conuulsions, specially in that part afflicted, which caused me to iniect into the wound oile of Terebinthinæ, with a little of the powder of Euphorbii, and of Aqua vitæ q. s. These were gently boiled togither, vntil the Aqua vitæ was consumed: and likewise I did imbrocate and annoint his thigh with the oiles of Cowslips, Lillies, and Chamamell, which did also greatly comfort and fortifie the greeued part. And thus within the space of fower and twenty howers, his cramps and conuulsions ceased. Now as I haue said, I do not heere set downe this annotation or obseruation of vainglorie, to the intent to blaze abroad the greatnes of the cure: but for that I would not conceale so fearfull a danger, & the way also how I preuented & cured it. Notwithstanding good reader, these accidents happened vnto this man, contrarie to the rules of my experience, yet I haue healed diuers fistulas with ẏ same medicines, & neuer saw the like troubles to happen, though the fistula were in the ioints with corruption of the bones, and likewise in other parts of the body, & seldom failed in the curing of any, vnlesse it were vpon those disordered persons, who refused to endure some paines, and a little restraint of libertie: for which causes I do heere aduertise all yong practisers in surgerie, not to intermeddle with any such, whatsoeuer they be, but I say with *Calmetius*, as desperate cures giue them ouer, and apply no hands vnto them: and although I haue heere set downe meete and conuenient remedies for the cure of a fistulas vlcer generally, with good and happie successe, neuertheles my meaning is not heer to binde any man to this order of curing only, but I wish al men to folow those approued remedies & waies of curing, which to themselues are best knowen, and haue found the most good by them: and not to be too much addicted to euery newfangled and strange inuention: for I say, new medicines make not a new art: for one good medicine well approued and experienced, is worth a number of some, which are indeed no better but as it were stumbling blocks to many yong practisers in the art. *Tagaltius* saith, wheresoeuer you set your mind, or wheresoeuer you cast your eies, a multitude of good remedies proffer and present themselues, wherein is excellently to be commended the diligence of our elders, and much more the affection they had to do good, whose labours are to be imitated, that in the wonderfull scope and varietie of things, left nothing vnapproued: all things done exactly and singularly wel considered of in writing, which now are committed to vs to take al the profit and commoditie, to wit, other mens trauels, an infinite number

[Margin notes: "Nota." beside "the extremity of the working…" and beside "tion: for I say, new medicines…"]

" ber of remedies were gathered, and now are left, and no account made
" of, bicauſe they be not cared for: but now adaies a little ſaluatorie diui-
" ded, with a few places or cels is ynough, alſo a ſillie plaiſter boxe, and
" this good man is content with a ſalue or two, which forſooth he taketh for
" an oracle, and thinketh it not méete to be controlled, &c. Thus briefly I end this hiſtorie or obſeruation, the which I haue recited onely for example ſake, that other Surgeons alſo might be prepared to do the like cure: ſo leauing the true cenſuring thereof, vnto the wiſe conſideration of the curteous and friendly reader.

The cure of a certaine ſoldier that was ſhot through the leg, and fractured the great bone called *Os Tibiæ*, or *Forſcilla maior*, this wound fell to Gangræna within two daies, by reaſon of a woonderfull inflammation that followed, he hauing alſo a very full and plethorick body.

Cap. 9.

This ſoldier was of a hot, cholericke, and furious nature: his body ſo repleniſhed with euill humors, that the parts about the Gangræna were maruellouſly inflamed, which greatly increaſed the furie and ſpreading of his gréefe, ſo that forthwith I was driuen to ſcarifie the afflicted part, with déepe ſections and ſcarifications, and alſo I opened with my launcet, all the ſmall vaines, which did appéere about the Gangræna: but where horſe léeches may be had they are very profitable to be applied, or for want of the horſe léeches, to open the ſmall vaines with a launcet is auailable: yet I ſuppoſe there is nothing better than the léeches, bicauſe they ſucke & draw out the aduſted and burnt bloud, which is congealed and compact in the vaines and places inflamed, then I fomented the corrupt parts twice a day with this Lixinium, which did ſtay the furie, and excellently clenſe and conſume the filthines and corruption.

A Lixinium. Am.Parc.

℞. Aceti optimi lib.j.
Mellis Roſ.℥.iiij.
Sir.Acetoſi ℥.iij.
Salis com.℥.v.

Boile all theſe togither, and then adde thereto
Aqua vitæ lib.ß.

When

When the corrupt part was herewith well fomented and bathed, then I applied vpon it Vnguentum Ægyptiacum after this deſcription following,

Vnguentum Egyptiacum

℞. Floris æris
Aluminis
Mellis com. } ana. ℥.iij.
Aceti acerrini ℥.v.
Salis com. ℥.j.
Vitrioli Rom. ℥.ß.
Sublemat. pulueriſati ʒ.ij.
Miſce & fiat vnguentum ſecundum artem.

Thus with pledgets of lint I did apply vnto the corrupt part, and vpon the ſame this Cataplaſma which is greatly commended by *Fallopius.*

A cataplaſma Fallopii.

℞ Rapum vnum domeſticum,
Vnam ſatis craſſam radicum Raphani,
Let them be ſcraped and ſufficiently cleanſed, then ad
Pulueris ſeminis ſinapis ℥.j.
Gariophillorum ʒ.iij.
Olei ſeminis lini
Olei micum iugland, vetuſtiſſimi } ana.q.s.

Let theſe be labored in a morter to the forme of a plaiſter or Cataplaſma, and then vſe it &c. Moreouer, there was applied about the mortified parts, thrée or fower times double this defenſiue, which is of a maruellous good operation, for it comforteth the member, and will not ſuffer it to receiue corruption.

A defenſiue. Vigo.

℞ Olei roſ. ex oliuis immaturis
Olei myrtini } ana. ℥.iiij.
Succorum plantaginis
& Solani } ana. ℥.ij.

Let all theſe be boiled till the iuice be conſumed, then ſtraine them, and adde thereto,

Ceræ albæ ℥.j.ß.
Farinæ fabarum
Farinæ lentium
Farinæ hordei
Sandalorum omnium } ana. ʒ.j.ß.
Boli Armeniaci ℥.j.
Pul. myrtyllorum
Granorum & foliorum eius } ana. ʒ.j.
Miſce.

By these means afore rehersed, the Gangræna was staied, in which time and space, I opened the liuer veine, and his body was also purged with Diacatholicon, and at sundry times we did giue him to eate of fine Mithridate, a little quantitie at a time, which as *Tagaltius* saith, is maruellous good to defend the filthie venemous fumes from hurting and offending the hart, which venemous vapours commonly ascende vp from the corrupt member: during all which time, he was adioyned to a thin and cooling diet. So after that the Gangræna was by these meanes fully and wholy staied, then the eschars were after remooued and taken away by these remedies next ensuing.

Vnguentum Tetrapharmacon. Galen.

℞ Picis nigræ
Resinæ
Ceræ
Adipis vaccinæ } ana. q.s.
Misce.

I say I did take of this said vnguent ℥.iiij. and of Vnguentum populeon simplex, ℥.iij. whereunto I did adde the yelks of two egs: all which togither were well laboured in a morter, I did heere with remoue the eschars, which being done, the part afflicted was after perfectly mundified with this excellent vnguent,

A mundifieng vnguent.

℞ Terebinthinæ claræ ℥.iiij.
Mellis rosati colati ℥.ij.
Succi plantaginis
Succi apij, } ana. ℥.j.

Let them boile vnto the consumption of the iuice, then take them from the fire, adding these heere vnder written, viz.

Vitellorum ouorum numero ij.
Farinæ hordei
Farinæ fabarum } ana. ℥.j.
Misce.

And after the place was heerewith well mundified and clensed: I did incarne & heale it vp with my incarnatiue vnguent, being mixed with Alumen combust. and also at sundry times I vsed Vnguentum ceraseos, paruum Mesuæ: and truly it is a very excellent incarnatiue.

Vnguentum Ceraseos paruum. Mesuæ.

℞ Aristolochiæ
Ireos
Sanguinis draconis
Hammoniaci
Sarcocollæ } ana ℥.j.
Lithargirij læuigati ℥. v.
Olei lib.j.

And

And likewise I used this plaister following alwaies upon the foresaid unguent untill the end of the cure.

Emplastrum nigrum.

℞ Olei rosſ.li.iiij.
Ceræ albæ lib.ß.
Minij lib.ij.
Camphor.℥.ß.

Boile togither your Minium and oile till it be blacke, then put in your ware, and last your Camphor: and thus within the space of ten wéekes he was safely cured, and his bone was againe united and knit, his splints and roulers were also taken away, and the plaisters which did remaine about his legge for the curing of the fractured bone were likewise remoued. And thus I finished this cure so effectually, as though he had neuer receiued hurt: but if the Gangræna should yet haue increased as oftentimes I haue séene, notwithstanding these and such like good remedies: then the last helpe would haue béene most miserable, that is, to cut off the corrupt member in the whole and sound parts, &c.

A necessarie note and obseruation for the cure of one master *Bucland*, dwelling at the signe of the George in Reading, a towne in Barkshire: he receiued a puncture or prick into the sinew or nerue of his right arme, by a most impudent and ignorant blood letter, which did pricke the sinew in steed of the liuer vaine. Cap. 10.

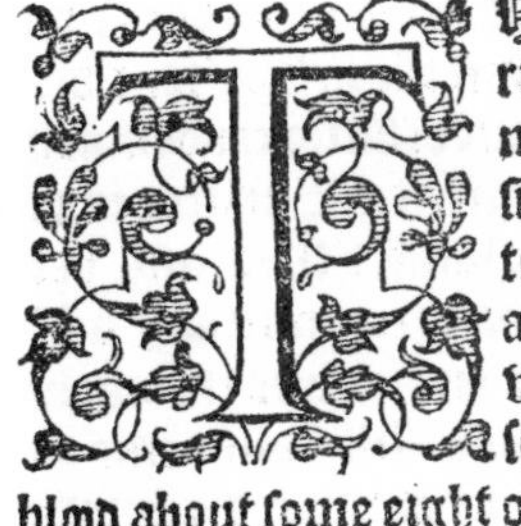

His master *Buckland* hauing a full and plethoricke body, and thereupon inclined to sicknesse: made his iourney unto Londō, only to take Physicke, which he did by the counsell of master Doctor *Simons*, who was in times past one of his olde acquaintance and familiar friends. After his body was well prepared and purged, the Doctor prescribed him farther remedie by a bill to be let blood about some eight ounces on the liuer vaine, appointing him thereunto also a Surgeon dwelling in this citie called master *Morland*. But (as he said) fortune owing him despite, by chance that Surgeon was not to be found, being called otherwise about some speciall cures: and therefore it was thought his comming home to be uncertaine: with that a friend of master *Bucklands*, who came to visite him and after spéeches had, understanding that he wanted a Surgeon to let him blood, said: If it it please you I will send for one that I do partly knowe, which is not onely a good Surgeon, but for letting of blood and drawing of a tooth, he is supposed to be as skilfull, as any man in this towne. Now such a one (said he) that can do so well in letting of blood, I would willingly heare of, and if it be your pleasure, I will sende my man for him in your name: in fine, a bad thing was easie to finde, for he was presently brought: then Master *Buckland* as you haue heard, being the sicke patient, deliuered vnto this bragging tooth drawer, and blood letter, the Physitians bill, which was written in English, but he answered and said, truly I can neither write nor reade: neuerthelesse, doubt you nothing but I can and will do it, as well as any man whatsoeuer, I dare make that comparison, quoth he: so the patient did reade the bill vnto him, which did signifie, that there should be eight ounces of blood taken from the liuer vaine on the right arme. Ho the liuer vaine sir (said he) I know it as well as all the Physitions and Surgeons in London: and so without any longer detracting of time, he went about his busines, and did so verub and chafe his arme, as though he had been laboring about horse heeles, and then bound his arme after his owne maner and fashion: all which being accomplished in the twinckling of an eie, or turning of a hand, this odde blood letter (as he called him) did without all regard or skill, vnaduisedly ouershoote himselfe, and thrust the said *Buckland* into the sinew in steed of the liuer vaine: then presently by the reason of the great sensibilitie and feeling of the prickt sinew, he fainted and sounded downe right, and much adoo they had to keepe life in him, so they gaue him presently to drinke Aquæ vitæ, and were further constrained, to burne a carde being folded vp round, and offered the smoke thereof into his nostrils: this done, he was laid vpon his bed, then al those that were about the sick patient, did begin to find great fault with his basenes, and want of skil, & condemned his handy worke: Well said he, I pray you be content, the matter is as much as nothing, for I haue had diuers that haue fainted thus, and yet were presently well againe: but the fault that I haue committed I will confesse, is for that the orifice was made too little, and indeede the onely cause was in your selfe, for that you did not hold still your arme as you should haue done: Then one of the standers by answered, a blinde shift is better than none at all, you might as well haue said, that he had eaten his horse, bicause his saddle lieth vnder his bed: Well said he, you speake merily, I know that saying hath been vsed as a iest for a long time, neuertheles by Gods helpe, I will make him well againe vpon my credit within twise foure and twentie houres: to be short, his words were but winde, for within that time and space, he had most of

Ignorance engendreth error.

The more the woorse.

these

these accidents which threatned great danger, for the wound had entertained and receiued many euill humors with extreme paines, inflammation, also a feauer, shiuering and rauing, and at certaine times conuulsions. Then they consulted togither, & determined to stay no longer upon this foolish coûterfet bloodletter his vain promises, for which cause they sent for D. *Simons*, and after his comming, it was strange for him to see such a sudden alteration: demanded of them what the cause might be: Then briefly they deliuered unto him all the euill that had happened, and the author and causer thereof: in the meane time I was also sent for: but here omitting other speeches had, I requested of them, that without tarrying I might lay all naked and bare. There I found the patient to haue all those euill Symptomes and accidents before rehearsed, and nature thereby greatly feebled and weakened. Then Doctor *Simons* called for the fellow that had so abused him: he being nothing ashamed of the matter, said here am I, what is your wils: You haue not beene circumspect, quoth Doctor *Simons*, in all things which concerne the methodicall perfection of this your handie worke: I will answer what I haue done, sir, quoth he: Then said the Doctor unto him, what reason had you, not onely to cômit a maruellous ouersight in pricking of the sinew, but also almost as foule a fault in stopping or closing up of the orifice of the wound, or pricke of the sinew, which now by your unskilfulnes is hidden under the skin, that at the very first you ought with all your industrie and diligence to haue kept open: Well, said he, I haue applied thereunto those medicines, which cannot be bettered, and are by me well approued to be good, either for pricks, or cuts of tendous sinewes, or vaines, but yet did I neuer see accidents thus secretly steale into a wound. I pray you what be your medicines, or remedies that you haue used, which are so good, and haue so euill successe: I tell you (said he) they are no beggerly medicines, but the best I could buie for my monie, the one is Gratia Dei, and the other is an Indian balme, which I know is good: for well I wot it cost me halfe a crown an ounce at the first hand: Your remedies (said I) may be profitable as they are used, although not for such pricks of sinewes: What is your reason I pray you (said he) I neuer heard any man say so but you: Quoth I, bicause at the beginning of all pricks of sinewes, you ought not to use either conglutinatiues or incarnatiues, untill the wound be past all danger of accidents, and then such medicines which haue propertie to incarne, and to couer the sinew with flesh may safely be used, neither are such wounds restored againe by balmes, according to the first intention, but onely in fleshie parts: Then he answered againe and said, you make here a greater stir before the patient and his friends than there is cause, for what though he be a little faint, he shal be well again by Gods grace, if he will be ruled by me but a little while: and I will stand to it for all your talke, it is but a small pricke onely in the skin: but admit the sinew were cleane cut asunder, which is I suppose a worse & more dangerous thing than the prick of a sinew, and yet (said he) without comparison or praise of my selfe I speake it, I haue without all this busines cured them when I had no such ouerseers or counsellers but my selfe alone: Why (said I) do you not thinke that a prick in the sinew is more dangerous, than that sinew which is cleane cut asunder: No (said he) you shall neuer make me beleeue, that a pricke by a small pointed thing, as is a launcet or a needle, can be so dangerous, as that which is cut asunder by a razor or knife, or other sharpe weapons: Now truly said I, I may well credit you in good sooth, that you can neither write nor reade, neither yet haue you any good experience: for if you had, you would neuer thus besot your selfe with such rude iudgements and fond opinions. Then he did begin as it were to open the gates of infamie, as is the maner of such shamelesse persons, specially against an expert and skilfull Surgeon of this citie of London, maliciously charging him that he had spoiled a Gentlewoman in the countrie, who hauing as this slanderer said, but a little pricke with a needle onely in the skin, and was in the ioint of hir fore finger of hir right hand, & by that small prick in the skin, she lost the vse of hir finger, which cure (said he) hath vtterly discredited him both with the Gentlewoman & hir friends: I answered & said, that might haue been any other mans cause, & I told him that my selfe haue known the like successe to happen in the cure of men of good iudgement, knowledge and experience, and yet in mine opinion, no fault or error at all committed by them, touching the right method and maner of curing such wounds in the skin, and other sundry parts: Well (said he) speake what you please, I do know the pricke with a needle in the skin is nothing so dangerous as you make it, in any body whatsoeuer, but it is said (quoth he) to be your maner that are Surgeons of London to hide and excuse one anothers fault, and to speake against such as I am, bicause I am a stranger, and none of your Companie, and therefore I am despised, and my medicines dispraised: Why (said I) euerie honest man, and faithfull true artist, that is diligent in his studie, and thereby attaineth to knowledge and skill, according to that measure which God of his great goodnes hath indued him with: such men we say are our brethren, and do accept them as good members of our Companie, whersoeuer they dwell and abide: but contrariwise, intruders, deceiuers, braggers and boasters, and such shamelesse shifters as your selfe is, which without either reason or skill, do abuse the art, and spoile the people, we exclude such

He hath moe fellowes that will point at other mens faults and imperfections, but forget their own.

It were good if it were so.

such bad persons cleane from us, and do account you all a sort of caterpillers and cosoners, not worthie to liue in the countrie and common wealth. Then I proceeded to his former speeches, as touching the pricke of a needle in the skin, and I said unto him: sith you will not beleeue me that such pricks are dangerous, I will shew you what *Tagaltius* saith, being a learned man in Physick and Chirurgery. He citing *Galen* in the first booke of his method, whose words in effect are these: Imagine one " come to us who hath but only a prick in the skin with a needle, that man " for the good disposition of his body may easily be cured, and to follow his " accustomed busines, hauing the part naked and bare, and without any " medicine at al, and yet receiue no hurt: but if he haue a full & plethorick " body, or a body of an il constitution called Cachochimicum in such a bo- " dy, the prick of a needle in the skin is hard to be cured. Then this proud boasting bloodletter who also would be Chirurgus chirurgorum, answered againe iustifieng his foule actions: I care neither for *Galen*, nor the other man you speake of, he meaning *Tagaltius*, for (said he) I haue done as good cures as the best of them both, & yet I hear they were a couple of good workmen: Then said the doctor, I am ashamed of thy impudency & beastly boldnes, and so for that cause he sharply reprehended him, & commanded him to auoide the place and presence of the patient: Then with unseemely behauiour & rude speeches which are unworthy the rehearsal, he departed &c. Now before I come unto the cure of the said puncture or pricke of the sinew, you shall first understand that the matter was so stopped in, that it could not by any meanes conueniently breath out, neither was there any easie passage for the medicines to go in: and therefore I did open the skin by incision directly upon the prick of the sinew, which I made of a sufficient length, that the matter which was stopped in, might the more freely and easily issue out, and that matter which did continually flow forth, was somewhat cleere, thin, and glutinous: like as though it had beene a slime or muscilage. Then I applied upon the said puncture or prick to mitigate the paine, these oiles following made first actually hot, which I used continually untill the aforenamed accident was remoued and taken away.

Note the rude answer of this proud bosting bloodletter.

Clowes.

℞ Oleorum Cham.
& Lumbrici } ana. ℥.ß.
Olei Euphorbij ℨ. j. ß.
Olei ex vitellis ouorum ℨ.ij.
Aquæ vitæ q.s.
Misce.

Since the time of this cure I found the like profit for appeasing of pains, in the cure of a womã, which also was prickt into the sinew: unto whom

whom I vsed these oiles following in the same order as the other afore rehersed.

℞ Olei Terebinthinæ
Olei Rosarum
Olei Lumbricorum
Olei Vitellorum ouorum } ana. ℥.iij.
Misce.

After I had (actually hot) applied the foresaid oiles, then I ministred therewithall, for the more securitie and spædie helpe to appease the paines, this worthy remedie which is described by *Vigo*.

Vigo. ℞ Medullæ panis & lactis vaccinæ confectæ cum oleis ros. & Chamæmeli cum vitellis ouorum & cum croco ana.q.s.

Boile all these togither vnto the thicknes of a plaister, the which I applied warme vnto the said puncture: also vpon this medicament, and likewise round about the whole member where any paine or inflammation was, this excellent cataplasma following.

Valeriola. ℞ Farinæ fabarum
Hordei
Lentium
Lupinorum } ana. ℥.iij.
Farinæ seminis lini
Fenugræci } ana. ℥.ii.
Farinæ orobi ℥.i.
Croci ʒ. ii.
Bulliant farinæ cum aceto & mel paruo.
fiat Cataplasma.

Also I haue vsed in the like cure done of late, this plaister following with great profit and ease vnto the patient,

℞ Radic.althææ
Farinæ hordei
Farinæ fabarum
Farinæ lentium. } ana.q.s.

Coquantur cum sapone, vel Lixinio barbitonsoris, whereunto you shall adde.

Wecker. Olei Rosarum
Olei Chamæmelini &
Olei Anethini } ana. q. s.
Also,
Terebinthinæ &
Croci paruum
Misce, & fiat Emplastrum.

I haue thought it not amisse here to giue you to vnderstand, that *Guido* doth admonish vs, not to vse at all those poultises which are wont to cure inflammations, for that such remedies in this cure, do rather putrifie and waste away the sinewes &c. And sith the chiefest thing in curing wounds of the sinewes is to appease the paine: therfore I haue thought it good here to set forth such chosen medicines as my selfe haue approued, for the better directing of those yong students, which haue not bin practised in the like maner & order of curing. Moreouer, whereas *Guido* with others do wisely declare that conuulsions are euill, & for the most part incurable, yet it so pleased God by these remedies heereafter set downe, he was in reasonable time & space quite deliuered of that euil accident, by annointing morning and euening all the hinder parts of his neck, and both his shoulder blades, and so downe all the spine of his back, euen vnto the hips with this vnguent,

℞. Olei Castorei ℥.j.
Olei Iuniperi ℥.ß.
Olei Liliorum &
Olei Vulpini } ana.ʒ.vj.
Misce.

This being accomplished as is before declared, then I proceeded from time to time, vntil the finishing of this cure, the which was done in the end with that most excellent Balme that I first obtained of the Lord of Aburgauenny, and (as is supposed) collected by M. *Hall* late Chirurgion of Maidenstone in Kent, and now by me brought into practise with diuers Chirurgions of London, and heere published in this booke: and I vsed the said balme with this vnguent following,

℞ Ceræ ℥.v. — Vnguentum aureum.
Resinæ quar.j.
Terebinthinæ lib.j.
Mellis quar. ß.
Mastiches
Thuris
Sarcocollæ
Myrrhæ
Aloes
Croci } ana.ʒ.ij.
fiat Vnguentum.

This approued vnguent and the aforesaide Balme togither, brought very speedily flesh vpon the hurt sinew: and hauing left the vse of the Cataplasma, then I did wrap the whole member round about cum Emplastrum Diachalcitheos, dissolued in Oleo rosarum & Lumbricorum,

corum, which did greatly strengthen the weake member: and thus with Gods helpe, by this maner of method and way of curing, he was restored againe to his former health &c.

The cure of a certaine stranger, which was wounded or thrust through his thigh with a Rapier, by one of his owne countrey men, being combating and fighting togither: the cure thereof was somwhat hard and difficult, by reason he was farther touched with *Lues venerea*, before he receiued his wound. Cap. 11.

Immediately after he had receiued his wound or thrust through his thigh, I was sent for vnto this cure, the patient lying at a strangers house in the Crouched Friers: yée shall héere note that he had a very strong, fat and corpulent body, and so a very big thigh: he was a man about thirty yéeres of age, all which being considered concerning the state and strength of his body, and the greatnes of the place wounded: then for the cure thereof I did ordaine a Flamula made of fine Lawne, the which was dipped in Oleo hyperici cum gummo and with a néedle made of Whale bone fit for such purposes, I did draw the said Flamula through the wound, and did leaue both the ends thereof hanging forth at the orifices of this wound, putting also a small tent in the dependant or lowest part of the wound, and the largest orifice which was at the inside of his thigh, and there it did rest for the space of two daies, applying also therto for the staying of the blood *Galen* his powder: and aboue the wound I laid a very good defensiue: after I did rowle it vp according to art. The second day at night he did require me to dresse him againe, for bicause the night before he said he was troubled with a feuer, as he supposed it to be, & so was perswaded by others, and for that cause he entertained a Phisition a countreyman of his, for to cure his ague, and also to sée his wound: Now when the wound was opened, it was without tumor or any other euil symptome, only I found a bloody sanies: for that cause I vsed next with the Flamula a very good digestiue, the which I dipped in Oleo rosarum, & melle rosar. ana. q.s. & so left the vse of oile of Hypericon. Then the next day in the morning, he complained of extreme paine which he had suffered all that night: then I opened the wound, and I did find as aforesaid, where with he

was

was somwhat disquieted in his body and mind: Then I drest him again, and he was very quiet and well all that day, and at night the wound tended towards digestion, which was (me thought) very well to be liked of: but the next day in the morning it was worse than before, a stinking bloody sanies, and the next day at night the matter was indifferent, yet in the morning by no means I could procure concoct and digest matter: notwithstanding the best digestiues and other good medicines I vsed. So the Phisition and the rest of his countrimen thought somewhat amisse in me, for that the patient his wound did heale and prosper no better: and in like maner I thought somwhat in the Physition, for that he could not find out the reason and cause of his supposed feuer. To come to the purpose, at the next opening in the presence of his Host of the house where he did lie, which was his interpretor, I desired him to demaund of the patient, when and where his paines did most afflict and trouble him, he answered in the night time and chiefly in his head, and also in his shoulders, legs, and armes, all which were very sore greeued and tormented: then I was bolder to procéede in examination, and asked him, if he had any breakings out in som particular parts of his body, he answered no, but onely a few scabs in his head, the which he did not perceiue, but since he was hurt and kept in his bed: and further he said he was very sore gréeued with the Hemorroides or piles, which for the basenes of the place, he said he was vnwilling to acquaint any mã with. Then I plainly told him he was touched with the French disease, so I being loth to giue offence said little more at that time, bicause I perceiued he had my words in disdain, vntil he considered better with himself: & against my next comming, he caused the Physition to méete with me: so after he had also séene and heard the whole matter, he likewise confirmed my sayings, that certainly it was the disease aforesaid: Why said the patient to the Doctor, doth our countrey yéeld such fruit & I being no Frenchman: He answered, God in his iustice plagueth most part of the world with that disease onely for sin & wickednes: so order was taken by vs presently, & we entred him into cure for that sicknes: but héere you shall vnderstand, that in all this time I did neuer alter or change mine intention of curing, neither did I leaue of the vse of the Flamula, vntill the wound was perfectly digested, which we could by no meanes procure vntill he was entred sixe daies in the diet, then altogither I left of digestiues and the vse of the Flamula, and vsed but short tents with good iniections, and also very often Oleum hyperici, with other conuenient remedies méete for this cure, which I haue plentifully published in this booke.

There were neither Hemorroids nor piles, vnder his correction but the F.P.

The cure of two Seafaring men which fell sicke at the sea of the Scorby. Cap. 12.

I Can not héere well passe ouer this briefe note or obseruation of the curing two seafaring men, which trauelled a long time vpon the seas, and there fell sicke of the Scorby, which infection as I gathered by inquiry, was reputed principally vnto their rotten and vnholsome victuals, for they said their bread was musty and mouldie Bisket, their béere sharpe and sower like viniger, their water corrupt and stinking, the best drinke they had, they called Beueridge, halfe wine and halfe putrified water mingled togither, and yet a very small and short allowance, their béefe and porke was likewise, by reason of the corruption therof, of a most lothsome and filthy taste and sauor, insomuch that they were constrained to stop their noses, when they did eate and drinke thereof: moreouer their bacon was restie, their fish, butter and chéese woonderfull bad, and so consequently all the rest of their victuals: by meanes hereof, and likewise lacke of conuenient exercise, cleane kéeping and shift of apparell, and againe, being in an ill disposed climate, and want of good aire: these causes and such like were the onely meanes they fell into the Scorby, for their gums were rotten euen to the very roots of their téeth, and their chéekes hard and swolen, their téeth were lose néere readie to fall out, their iawes very painfull, their breath of a filthy sauor, that at what time I drest their gums, and washed their mouthes, the sauor was so odious, that I was scarse able to staie and abide it: in like maner their legs were féeble, and so weake, that they were scarse able to carrie their bodies: moreouer, they were full of aches and paines, with many blewish & reddish staines or spots, some broad and some small like flea bitings, or the graines of a Pomegranate, likewise their legs were colde, hard, and swolen, which caused me to fear a Gangræna, for coldnes in such extremities being in corrupt bodies full of euill iuice, doth challenge putrifaction, which disease or sicknes, although it be in some safely cured, yet experience daily prooueth that a number also die. Now the first thing that required helpe by Chirurgery was their gums, and their legs, being the conioined cause, but for that I will procéede as orderly as I can in my writing, I will begin with the antecedent cause inwardly, which was done and performed by the aduise and counsell of learned Physitions, who very confidently set me down their opinions for their maner & order of purging, with other remedies, as hereafter followeth: First as I said, euacuation going before, to diminish the humors sore abounding, it was therfore thought most méete to begin with blood letting in the middle vain on the left arme, & I did then take from ech of them vij. or viij. ounces of blood. The next day following they were also well purged with this purgation, ℞. Diasenæ ʒ.j.ß. Sirr. fumariæ, ℥.j. Aquæ scabiosæ, ℥.iij. Misce. and herewith they were purged. Also euerie seuenth or eight day they were likewise purged with the pils of Fumitorie ʒ.j. made into fiue pils, so as I say, after they were well purged, then in the meane space, there was prepared for them in a readines this drinke following, which continually they did drinke at their meales, and also as often as they were desirous to drinke. The order and making thereof is thus: first there must be prepared a cleane vessell of eight gallons, which was filled full of new ale, and then was added to it of Coclearia or Scorby grasse a pecke, being purely picked, and cleane washed, and also brused in a stone morter, and after put into the vessell with the ale, then was added thereto of long Pepper ℥.j. Cinnamon and Ginger of each halfe an ounce, of Saffron ʒ.ij. all these spices were put into a fine linnen cloth or bag, and so hanged in the ale, with the herbes aforesaid, and thus it rested two daies before they did drinke of it. And further it is to be remembred, that euery morning they did eate a messe of this Almond milke being newly made, and it did them very much good. ℞. two spoonefuls of French barly, and séeth it in a reasonable quantitie of running water till it be soft, then adde to it of Almonds blaunched ij. ounces, then take of this liquor a pound, and put to it of Coclearia or Scorby grasse, Fumitorie, and water Cresses, of each halfe a handfull, but first mixe with the Almonds in the beating, of this liquor, for feare the Almonds will turne to an oile, then boile all togither to the consumption of the third part, then adde to the straining, of fine Sugar ℥.j.ß. of Rose water ℥.ij. let all these séeth a little, and then reserue it to your vse: In like sort euerie euening towards fower of the clocke they did drinke a good draught of posset ale, whereunto was added of the iuice of Scorby grasse a spoonfull, with a little of the powder of Cinnamon and some Sugar, and now and then in stead thereof a good draught of Wormwood wine. Their meates that they did eate was Mutton boiled, and somtimes Veale and chickens, &c. seasoned with veriuice made of grapes, and thickened with ote meale, or the crums of white bread, with a few Currans, and Raisons of the sunne. Moreouer, there was added of Scorby grasse, Fumitorie, water Cresses, and Soldanella. Their bread was made of the finest wheate, and of a day old. Now héere note you well, that euerie day or second day, one hower after they had receiued a certaine fume, the description héere-after

Blood letting.

The purgation. D.D.

A drink good for the Scby. G.R.

Almond milk. G.R.

after followeth, then they did presently drinke of the aboue named Almond milke. And after their sweating was ended, I did immediately bathe their legs: which done, I annointed them, and lastly I applied a plaister, which hereafter shall be also nominated. Now for that their gums were so exceeding stinking and rotten, I did at the very beginning scarifie their gums with a fleame, then presently I did as it were touch, or wipe their gums gently ouer with a certaine blewish water, which the goldfiners haue used for refining their golde, and haue themselues no use for it, the force and strength being by them greatly consumed and wasted: for the which cause it is called the weake water. After the use hereof, I did cause them certaine times in the day and in the night, to gargarise or wash their gums and mouthes with my lotion published in my booke for the curing of *Lues Venerea*, Cap. 6. Whereunto many times I mixed the sirr. of Mulberies, q.s. also I did at sundrie times use of the afore named blewish water, and did take thereof ℥.ß. whereunto I did put of Plantaine water ℥.viij. and here with I did mundifie and clense their gums. Also it is knowen most certainly what great good is done in curing of such rotten gums and sore mouthes, onely with this gargarisme, which is published by *Iulius Palmerius*, & it is also set forth of late by master *Banister* in a booke, which he calleth his *Antidotarie Chirurgicall*, ℞. Hordei integri p.ij. Eupatorij, Nicotianæ, Plantaginis, Morscis gallinæ, Ros. rub. ana m.j. boile these togither in Aqua lib.iiij. till the one part be consumed, then adde thereto Mellis rosar. Sirr. rosarum siccarum ana. ℥.iij. Aluminis vsti, Calcanti vsti, ana. ℥.ß. boile all these with a walme or two, & so let it coole, and then keepe it to your use.

A very singular gargarisme.

Also I haue found great good by the use of this powder, which is published by that reuerend learned man *Wyerus*, who hath written most profoundly for the cure of the Scorby, take of salt and burne it in a crusible, whereunto ye shall adde of the powder of Pomegranate flowers, and so mixe them togither, & herwith I did many times rub well their gums. Moreouer, I haue in times past used Vnguentum Ægyptiacum, and also a powder called of some Puluis Alchimisticus, or Caput mortuum, it is the dead head, of Aqua fortis, I also after washed their mouthes with vineger and salt water, q.s. and by these meanes I haue cured manie sore mouthes specially in children, when I was Chirurgion unto the children in Christs Hospitall, where I haue had twenty, or thirty infected with the Scorby at a time. After I had well mundified and cleansed the mouthes and gums of these two men, then I did administer a certaine fume, by the aduice and counsell of D.D. which fume was receiued in at their mouthes by a funnell after this manner, I did take of Mirrhæ, Olibani, Assæ fætidæ ana. ℥.ij. Aceti vinaci lib.j. which gums were

I was Chirurgion of Saint Bartholomewes hospitall in Smithfield, and also of Christes hospitall for

were grosly beaten, then they were tied loosely in a fine linnen cloth, and so put into the viniger, then there was prepared an earthen pot fit for the purpose, well glassed or nealed, and at those times when it was to be vsed, there was prepared a funnell made fit in widenes and compasse vnto the mouth of the said pot, & so it was well passed or luted togither, with this lute called of *Schilander*, and many other good distillers and Alcumists *Lutum sapientiæ*, and it is proued very necessary to ioine and conglutinate two vessels togither seruing for distillations, or otherwise as afore said. ℞. Clay and Fullers haire, with whites of egs and sand, thus I ioined the pot & the funnel togither, and then I set it vpon a chafingdish of coles, and I let it boile gently, & then caused the patients to sit vp in their beds one after another, & so they receiued into their mouthes the fume or smoke, that passed forth of the top of the said funnell, & this was vsed diuers mornings before they did take their Almond milke, and also certaine times in the euening, and did sweate halfe an hower after it in their beds: which fume was administred most chiefly to open their obstructions inwardly, and so being well cooled and dried with warme clothes, they did rise out of their beds, and went to the bathing of their legs, and annointings as followeth, ℞. the flowers of Chamomell, Melilote and Wormewood, the leaues of Coclearia, Water Cresses, and Brookelime, of each a handfull, of the berries of Iuniper two handfuls, of Malmsey a quart, running water q.s. sweete butter a pound, these were boiled togither, to the consumption of the third part, which bath did bring out in a short time a number of spots, which before lay hid in the flesh, and herewith very warme, they were a long time togither bathed, with double woollen clothes of white cotton or baies, & then dried them very well, with hot linnen clothes: and as I haue before mentioned, they were presently annointed somtimes with Vnguentum Agrippæ, and somtimes with Vnguentum Brioniæ, or Dialthææ cum gum. and also their legs were all wrapped round with this plaister, ℞. Emplastrum Deminio lib.ij. Gummi Armoniaci lib.ß. being dissolued in Malmsey, then put them togither, adding thereto Axungiæ humani ℥.ii. ß. I boiled these togither to the forme of a plaister. I found also very much profit by the Cuminum plaister published in this booke. And thus by the helpe of God and carefull diligence, they were both perfectly cured, and diuers other persons of good account since that time, onely by this maner and order of curing aforesaid, &c.

certain yeers togither, till I was called to other speciall seruices.

The Fume. D.D.

The Bath.

Vnguents & plaisters.

The

The cure of a Lieutenant which was shot into the right buttock with a poisoned bullet. Cap. 13.

FRiendly Reader, amongst sundry other special cures which I haue noted, not onely in mine owne works and procéedings, but also in other mens of greater yéeres, antiquitie, and experience in the art of Chirurgery, this one cure following in my simple opinion and iudgement, is not to be passed slightly ouer and buried in forgetfulnes, if it were but in respect of the strangenesse and rarenes of such a cure, and of the good and happy successe that followed.

TO procéede to my purpose, the said Lieutenant was a man about the age of sixe and thirty yéeres, hauing a strong and able body answerable to his valor and corage, which appéered in his seruice against the enimie: he receiued a wound in his right buttocke by a bullet, being then (as he said) somwhat far off from the enimies fort when he was shot in and wounded, which bullet was so secretly lodged, that by no conuenient meanes possible at the first dressing, I could get knowledge or vnderstanding certainly where the shot should lie, by reason of the turning or folding of the muskles, and sensibilitie of the patients body, yet I would then very faine haue enlarged the wound by incision, whereby the better to haue come to the bullet, but the patient would in no wise suffer to haue it done: then I perceiued he was partly ouer wearied by the probation and searching, for that cause I thought it vaine to molest or disquiet the patient any longer at that time, but so I let him rest, sith it was his mind & desire till the next day, supposing no euill accidents would haue hapned, at the least wise in so short a time & space: and my reason that led me thus to thinke, was for that I did read how Lead had a certaine singularitie agréeing to nature, for which cause I preserued him at that instant time, with the oile of Whelpes, called Oleum catulorum, with defensatiues, and comfortable oiles and plaisters fit for that purpose, as I haue vsed to many others which were wounded with gun shot, especially in such fleshie places, where the oile is best to be vsed, and haue alwaies had therewith good lucke and happie successe, howbeit (contrary to expectation) within six houres after he was dressed, he did begin to haue a troubled minde, full of sorrowes and disquietnes: and complained much of his wound, how it did greatly molest him, and that with a strong kinde of pricking or biting, as if his wound

wound had béen laid in a bed of pricking or sharpe stinging nettles, and for that cause he would very willingly haue béen opened and new dressed againe: then I considered it was but two of the clocke in the afternoone when I preserued him first, therfore I told him, I hoped that his paines would cease without further trouble extraordinary, by reason of the benefit of those remedies which I had applied to him, and so I perswaded him to be quiet till the next day in the morning, neuertheles in the night season he was extremely handled, and very sore vexed with a sharpe and perilous feauer, and shiuerings without intermission or ceasing, his pulse great, swift and fast, so that oftentimes he fell into soundings, by reason of the anguish and paine, and did speake very idlely, coueting to lie groueling on his face, with other perilous signes and accidents. The morning approching, when the watch was discharged, and the ports opened, there was sent in haste a messenger, that imparted vnto me as you haue heard, what a lamentable and miserable case he was in that night, as though the whole member had béen torne with dogs, the which to heare did not a little trouble me, for I considered with my selfe that the captaines and other braue seruitors, as master *Crips*, lieutenant to sir *Phillip Sidneys* horsemen, master *Bowsfield*, master *William Harcote*, master *Barfoote*, & lieutenant *Browne*, with others, who had béen my patients, reposed a great trust and confidence in me, for which cause I did thinke it stood me vpon to be circumspect and warry, least I might get but little credit thereby. And bicause I woulde be loth to be ouertaken with vnskilfull rashnes, I desired the messenger to returne backe againe with spéede, and to intreat the patients friends that they would call some Physition or skilfull Surgeon, whom they thought good of, to be at his dressing, for I tolde him I suspected a Gangræna, and that was the cause of my long tarrying, till I had prepared all things in a readines for that purpose: in which time and space, they had brought vnto the patient a stranger, borne (as they said) in the east Countries, and being as it séemed of their acquaintance, which had many yéeres practised Physicke and Surgerie, somtimes in the enimies campe, and somtimes with the States, a man doubtles learned, and also of no lesse iudgement and practise in the Art of Surgery: he was giuen to vnderstand before I did come to the patient, how he was shot, and what euill accidents had hapned since his first dressing: in which time (as I haue said) I did ordaine such remedies which I supposed to be the best & most méetest for the cure of a Gangræna. But after spéeches had with him, he desired me before I did prepare any of my remedies for the dressing of the patient, that without staying I would take off all things from the wound, the which presently I did: and so all being laid open, the wound was found maruellously altered and changed, for it did looke in colour much like vnto ashes, or rather more wanner like vnto Lead, and the whole member very vnweldy and heauy, which were to me very strange, and extraordinary signes, such as I neuer did see happen in other common wounds made with gun shot: then he conferred with me and others that were present, and said by all signes and tokens, the bullet is poisoned with some venemous mixture, and assure your selfe that the danger is greater, and neerer at hand than you are aware of, and therefore said he, if you should follow that course you haue begun, and neglect the time, and so pretermit such knowne helpes, which I shall acquaint you withall, or the like in effect, the patient will hardly escape, for truly (said he) that which you haue done, sith they are no apt remedies for extraction and drawing out of venom and poison, it is all ministred and done in vaine: then I remembred that to vse vnapt & contrary remedies, was dangerous, specially in such causes, and therefore without delay in due time, I determined with my selfe to follow his counsell and direction, and to deale plainly. I suspecting mine owne knowledge in the cure of a poisoned wound made with gun shot, I thought it not best to attribute vnto my skill herein greater sufficiencie than was in me to performe: and sith it stood vpon the patients life, I did with all curtesie of speech and great thankfulnes towards him, so deale herein, that thereby I might become the more learned and expert in the cure of a poisoned wound made with gun shot, and so craued his further counsell in this cure: in which doing I did not thinke it any discredit or disgrace vnto me, seeing *Guido* a man of great knowledge and vnderstanding in Physicke and Chirurgery, as experience daily doth teach „ vs, saith, it is not possible for one man to haue all knowledge in himselfe, „ for one man may know that, which another knoweth not: To proceede, I must confesse he was as willing to shew me any thing he could pleasure me in, as I was desirous to craue it at his hands: he was like vnto some in these daies, which may be compared in nature and qualitie vnto *Timon* of Athens, being men fraught full of wrath and choler, and are alwaies more readier with malitious and enuious harts, and with curiositie of words, to deface, quarrell and contend with vncomely comparisons and scoffing speeches, and most bad behauiors behinde mens backs, as though others were abiects and reproches vnto the world, in respect of themselues, and their owne skils, when indeed they ought with concord and vnitie in a christian and brotherly loue, to bend their whole indeuor for the speedie recouery of their patients health, and credit of their brethren: but contrariwise (I say) argueth the lacke of a good conscience, howsoeuer they brag and boast of their owne exquisite knowledge in

Nota.

in the Art of Physicke and Chirurgerie. But to leaue such in their malice gnawing of their owne bones, and come againe to this skilfull Physition and Chirurgion aforesaid, who without further detracting of time, counselled me to make deepe incision, & then with a paire of Tenacles, crowes bils, and rauens bils, to take hold of the bullet, and to bring it out so easily as may be, then to scarifie well the lips or sides of the wound, which done, yee shall presently set on a strong cupping glasse on a flame of fire, that yee may the better euacuate and draw out the venemous and poisoned blood, which lurketh deepely in the bottome of the wound, whereby his paines may be the sooner asswaged. So vnderstanding herein all his whole meaning, neuerthelesse I did not take euerie word he spake for a gospell, till I had seene farther triall, but followed him so far as reason and experience did lead me: and I told him, though I had neuer seene a poisoned wound made with gun shot, and so had not cured any, yet I did reade in the writings of famous men of our time, that hardly or not at all, can a bullet of Lead receiue any venemous or poisoned mixture, but that the flame of the fire out of the peece doth extinguish and kill the force and strength of any poisoned shot: and also againe it is farther said, that those euill accidents do happen to wounds made with gun shot, partly by reason of the corruption of the aire, especially in hot and moist regions, for there the aire is most apt to increase putrifaction: and it is farther said, that southerly windes do increase putrifaction, insomuch that Butchers do refuse to kill flesh but for one day during the time: moreouer, such accidents do happen by reason of rotten and stinking mists, rising out of marish grounds, being neere sea coasts, & also from dead carkases, corrupt leistals & ditches, and where are multitude of people: especially in camps and great armies of men, many lothsome and stinking venemous vapors are ingendred, all which corrupt aires being receiued into their bodies that are wounded with gun shot, and so meeting with bodies that be of an ill disposition called Cacochimia, often times do so breede venemous and poisoned wounds. To this effect and such like words, as my memory serued me I spake vnto him: But he answered me againe, you speake I perceiue herein as your bookes lead you, but I tell you as experience hath often taught me, and it is no new or strange opinion. Then I considered they were very learned men that held both opinions, with long large discourses, as also sundry obiections of the one side and of the other: and sith the controuersie is amongst such great learned men, I will leaue it heere to their wise considerations.

Onely freindly Reader I must craue pardon for a litle digression, but I wil be short & so come againe to my purposed matter. As I haue said, I will

will not héere meddle with the state & condition of this controuersie as a controller of learned men, lest I should greatly wrong them, & vnawares defraud you of the truth: But this I must tell you, ỹ in séeking after the experience & proofe of this matter according to that gift which by Gods goodnes I attained vnto, I haue héerein confirmed my selfe: for not long since I being sent for to Portsmouth vnto the right honorable the Earle of Sussex, about the cure of master *Muns*, Lieutenant of the towne: who by misfortune receiued a great wound in his head. In the time of my abode there, I desired the master Gunner of the towne, that he would shew me that fauour, as to let me sée an arrow shot out of a Musquet: for I thought I could no way so wel come to the true knowledge of my desire, but by such martiall men, as were expert and well practised in such fiery engins so very courteously he granted my request, and I asked his opinion, if it were possible by his art and skill to poison a bullet of Lead: He answered that he did know that a bullet of Lead might be poisoned, & moreouer he said it is against the law of arms to shoot a poisoned shot: againe, it is present death if such shot be taken or found about any enimy. And I haue since heard it confirmed by diuers Captaines and old soldiers, who also haue said vnto me, that they did know them that were executed for the same. Now I come to the charging of his péece, which I did sée himselfe do, and he deliuered it to one of the soldiers of the towne, who presently did take his rest, and discharged the said péece against a gate, being distant from the place where he stood, about two hundred or eight score paces, and the arrow did stick very déepe in the post of the gate, where by force it was taken out, but we found not so much as one feather of the arrow touched with the flame or fire out of the péece. And although so manifest a truth néedeth no witnes, yet bicause there was at that present time in the towne with the Earle of Sussex a learned Physition called M. *Trip* of Winchester, which can witnes with me that I speak the truth héerin, who saw the arrow that was shot out of the péece, and I haue séene the like done in a Caliuer with our common sheafe arrowes. All this (me thinke) as I haue said, prooueth that much lesse doth the fire burne out the impression of a poisoned bullet if it be not able to burne the feathers of the arrow: for being charged, as I haue séen it, to my iudgement the arrow is gone out of the péece afore the flame of fire doth appéere in sight, or the report of the péece can be heard: And if it were so that the flame of fire should burne the feathers, I sée no reason why the arrow should be feathered at all: but I suppose euery man cannot shoot off an arrow and saue the feathers, yet I am perswaded, he that hath learned to poison a shot, hath also learned so to shoot it off, that it shall worke the mischiefe he purposeth. And now for that I woulde be loth to make a long and tedious discourse of that, wherin I haue had so small experience: I will therfore procéed vnto the order of the cure, that was this: I did presently as I was directed, make reasonable large & déep incision, which don, I did take out the bullet that lay somwhat déep, but by the way, it was (me thought) strange to sée the bullet flat and ragged of the one side, as if it had béen battered against a rough wall, and very round one the other side: and also manifestly séene certaine stabs in many places, as if it had béen the pricking of a dagger, neither caried it the color of other bullets: for it séemed as though the powder of rustie iron, gréene Copperas, or some glassie color had béene sprinckled or stained in the Lead: Then it was put into the fire, & being melted, these colors vanished away, but what maner of poison it should be, that I could not learn. After the bullet was taken out, and the edges of the wound scarified, I did set on a large cupping glasse, such as comprehended all the wound, and did mightily draw a good quantity of blood: then I would willingly haue vsed a bright cauterizing iron, bicause it was in a place it might be safely done without danger to the patient, for that the nature of fire, is to tame the malice and fury of venome and poison, all this he confessed may well be vsed, and it is allowed of many excellent men: But (said I) I haue found out by diligence a more safe and familiar remedie, which doth also make an eschar, but not like an actuall cauterie with so much paine, and moreouer it doth stay the venome from creeping vpwards, neither will it suffer the poisoned vapors to spread abroad, or enter into the noble or vnnoble parts, as to the hart by the arteries, or into the liuer by the vaines, or into the braine by the sinewes, and so consequently into all the rest of the parts and members of the bodie: then still héedily I followed his direction, and thought my selfe happy of such a conductor or leader, so I applied this his foresaid remedy, which truly wrought maruellous strangely and to great effect, and I filled the wound with pledgets dipped in the same very hot: and this is the composition and receit thereof now following,

A singular good remedie to destroy venome and poison. D.

℞. Olei sambucei ℥.j.
Olei Mirrhæ ʒ.ij.
Olei sulphuris ʒ.iij.
Spiritus vini q.s.
Misce.

And vpon the same was laid a broad plaister of Theriaca Andromicha, héere doubting the malicious crueltie and venositie of the said poisoned shot, for that cause it was thought good to vse twise togither the afore named sharpe medicine, immediately vpon the remouing of one

eschar

eschar after another, which eschar was taken away by this remedie following, which is wonderfull good to mollifie and digest the eschars, and also to cease the paines: this vnguent by negligence was omitted and left out in the former impression of this booke.

Vnguentum mollificatiuum which I vsed to remooue the eschars.

℞. Axungiæ humanæ
Anseris
Gallinæ
Medullæ ceruinæ } ana. ℥.ij.
Terebinthinæ lotæ in aqua vitæ ℥.j.
Ceræ q.s.
Misce,& fiat vnguentum secundum artem.

Now héere it is to be noted, that presently at his comming to this patient after he was dressed, he gaue him to drinke this preseruatiue,

A preseruatiue. D.

℞. Aquæ acetosæ ℥.iij.
Mithridati opt. ʒ.ß.
Sirr.de succo Limonium ℥.j.ß.
Diascordij ʒ.j.
Terræ Germanicæ ℈.ij.
Misce.

After the vse of these aforesaid remedies which were vsed at sundry times, about the first day this one accident happened, that aboue the rest I noted, which in my iudgement was very strange, that without any reasonable cause knowen, he had a number of foule & filthy stooles, full of corrupt excrements, as if it had béen the scrapings of leather, which also did weaken the patient, so that I supposed, his loosenes of body would haue caried him away vnto death. Then the Physition said he would not stop it, bicause it was the worke and benefit of nature. After the malignitie of this wound was by the foresaid remedies partly destroied, then I vsed these medicines following, which haue a great attractiue facultie, and did euacuate the virulent and poisoned matter, so that those which saw him in his great extremitie, being almost pined and ouerworne with paines and griefe, wondered and also reioiced at the greatnes of the successe,

An attractiue vnguent.

℞. Ceræ Citrinæ
picis naualis
Sepi ouini
Olei antiqui } ana.℥.iiij.
Galbani.℥.j.
Misce.

Héerewith sometimes I mixed Vnguentum Ægyptiacum, and so found it a very good medicine, and againe at other times I vsed it alone, and

and very often I used to mixe with it Mercurij præcipitati, and so dipped pledgets and tents of the same in Oleo hyperici, cum gummo all which did helpe to attract, digest, and suck out the venom, whereby the hurt part was greatly reuiued and comforted, and vpon these I applied an attractiue plaister, which doth sufficiently call backe the poison and venemous matter,

An attractiue plaister.

℞. Galbani
Ammoniaci
Bdellij
Sagapeni
Opopanacis } ana.℥.j.
Picis albæ ℥.iij.
Myrrhæ ℥.j.
Olibani ℥.ij.
Propoleos ℥.viij.
Magnetis ℥ ii.ß.
Olei Terebinthinæ, & Scorpiorum q.s.
Misce.

Thus I continued with these foresaid medicines till all the accidents were ceased, & so kept open the wound for a space, then I vsed other remedies for consolidation & restoring againe of the lost substance, which remedies I haue plentifully in this Booke specified for the cure of wounds made with gun shot.

And thus fréendly Reader yée shall vnderstand, I write not this obseruation in mine owne praise, but chiefly (as may appéere) for the good of my countrimen and countrey wherein I was borne and bred, so that they which will be carefull and diligent in spending of their time in labor and studie, not onely in reading of good authors, but also to endeuor themselues (as I haue before said) to be conuersant with learned Physitions, and well experienced Surgeons, for the better attaining vnto learning and knowledge, may in the end enioy the fruits of their labor and diligence: for idlenes yéeldeth as great profit, as a barren and dry trée good fruit. If any man be further desirous to be yet satisfied concerning the cure of a poisoned wound made with gun shot, let him reade *Iosephus Quercetanus*, a very learned writer in his booke of Gun shot, which is lately translated into English: and also read *Ioannes de Vigo*, without whom many of vs are often to séeke in our worke and practise, though in the cure of gun shot he was not so curious as som other, which indéed haue found out many excellent and approued remedies amongst the rest, for the cure of gun shot, &c.

The

The cure of a Pioner, which was shot into the left shoulder, so that the bullet lay secretly hid towards the chine or hollownes of the patients bodie, and also was shot through the secret parts, and so into his thigh, where I tooke out the shot. Cap. 14.

It happened that a certaine Pioner, whose name was *Barnard Thirkill*, borne in Yorke shire, seruing vnder master *Clifford*, an excellent enginer, and he himselfe vnder the conducting and leading of Generall *Norrice*, at the siege of Nemegham: this Pioner (as you haue heard) first receiued a wound with a bullet into his left shoulder, so that by reason of the vehemencie of the stroke, a breach was made in the bone, and there remained in the saide wound certaine shiuers or small péeces of bones troubling him greatly, with much paine and pricking. And though the wound was sufficiently inlarged when the bullet was taken out, yet could the shiuers by no meanes be altogither brought out, by reason they were strongly fastned vnto the flesh and pannicles, and the patient being a hot, cholerike and raging fellow, would not suffer me to cut them out: for which cause, the cure was thereby prolonged, and the accidents did grow much more troublesome, and great putrifaction did follow, and the blood, which at the first was clotted and congealed in the hollownes or bottom of the wound, could by no meanes possible be altered or turned into matter, notwithstanding, the best digestiues, and such like remedies, which I daily vsed to others: and the reason was as I gathered, by the paines and ouerlong lying of the small fragments and péeces of broken bones, which could not be apprehended or taken out with tennacles, crowes bils or rauens bils. And moreouer, for that the corruption and matter could finde no frée or easie passage, it had like to haue defiled part of the whole & sound bone, as we might plainly perceiue and sée: it is farther to be noted, that during al the time of his sicknes, he would in no wise take any Physick, not so much as a clister, or opening of a vaine, by meanes hereof, and other causes which hereafter shall be declared, impostume did rise vpon impostume, in such sort, that I was often driuen to make new incisions. But an other cause or reason there was, why the wound became so stubborne and rebellious, for that this rusticall borish fellow was of a maruellous dogged and churlish nature and disposition, and vsually giuen and delighted to drinke all sorts of strong drinks, in like sort he

would

would couet to eate bacon, salt béefe, hard chéese, salt butter, and dried fish if he could by any meanes come by it, and looke what was hurtfull unto him, therein he tooke his greatest pleasure and delight: and thus (as the common prouerbe goeth) he laid gorge upon gorge, ouercharging his stomacke with immoderate eating & drinking, saying unto me, this diet did greatly refresh him: insomuch that I was in despaire of his recouery, and many times repented me that euer I enterprised this beastly cure, by reason of the causes aforesaid, which oftentimes unluckily did fal out: againe, the naughtines of his disordered body was such, that his very sweats were noisom unto us, for he did smel extreme rammish, like unto a ranke bore or goate, but in the end he was brought to great debilitie and weaknes, and his gréedie stomacke almost cleane taken away: for which cause I was constrained to bethinke my selfe of these great lets and hinderances, and set apart all digestiues whatsoeuer, and did take me unto Ægyptiacum, which I used certaine times dissolued in this decoction, and iniected it into the wound,

He was also a very slouen and nastie.

℞. Aquæ hordei lib. ij.
Vini albi lib. j.
Mellis rosarum ℥. iiij.
Fol. plantaginis
Fol. & florum centauri minoris
Absynthij } ana. m. ß.

A very good decoction.

Boile these togither, to the consumption of the third part, and so reserue it to your use: somtimes I used this decoction alone, and somtimes I dissolued the Ægyptiacum in white wine and Aqua vitæ, and I filled the wound with pledgets dipped in the same, after it had béen oftentimes iniected: which being done, I laid ouer all the agréeued parts this poultis very well warmed, which did comfort him greatly,

℞. Neruale lib. iiii.
Fenegreeke ℥. iii.
Lineseede ℥. vi.
Barley meale
Beane meale } ana. m. i.

The Cataplasma of Neruale.

The powder of the roots of Marshy mallows being first dried, a handfull and a halfe, the floures of Cammomell and Melilot, being also well powdered of each a handfull, the leaues of Roses dried and powdered two handfuls, Saffron two scruples, the yelks of foure egges: first relent the neruale, which being done put in the rest one after another, continually stirring it: that being done, put in the yelks of egges in the cooling, when you use it for the like causes or els not, and so receiue it to your use, and it will be very hard and stiffe: and when you will occupie

H of

of it, take sixe, seuen or eight ounces more or lesse, as you haue occasion: if in cold causes, relent it ouer a chafing dish of coles, and put to it either Malmsie, Muskadell, or Sack, and in hot causes I haue often vsed white wine or milke: and for want of all these, I being at the seas and other places, I did take béer, and somtimes faire water, and so relente it gently togither, till it did come to the thicknes or body of a poultis, and beware of ouer boiling bicause of the egs: this poultis I euer caried with me both by sea and land, for it is very ready at all néedes, and it will last and continue a long time, and doth profit much. Now (as I haue before rehearsed) I did take of this poultis a conuenient quantity, and dissolued with it Malmsie q.s. & so very warm plaister wise, I applied it well ouer his shoulder, & it eased him greatly: & whereas before I was greatly in doubt he would haue giuen vs all an Vltimum vale, yet through the assistance of almighty God, with the meanes and helpe of the afore named remedies, those gréeuous accidents ceased, and the corruption thorowly clensed, and the smal fractured péeces of bones did lose and come away gently of themselues, and his stomack was againe restored, yet it was a long time before he was perfectly cured: for there did follow a certaine inflation, or puffing vp of cold, windy and waterish humors in his neck and shoulders, and so downe all his arme and hand on the same side where his hurt was: and therefore I was driuen after to bathe all the parts with this bath following.

Nota.

A bath.

Sea water lib.xii. Aqua vitæ lib.ii. I vse alwaies Sack in stéed of the Aqua vitæ, but it was not there to be had: the flowres of Cammomill, Melilot, Wormwood, and Dill, Fenell, Sage, Basill, Mints, Marieram of ech a handful: the séeds of Cummin, and Baiberies being brused, of ech two handfuls, for want I had not these herbes gréene, I did take most of them dried: and there was also put in a good fat shéepes head well chopped in péeces, which by ouer sight was left out in the former impression: all these were boiled to the consumption of the third part, and héerewith I bathed his neck, shoulder, arme, and hand, twise a day: so after the parts agréeued were well fomented and bathed, then presently I annointed him with these oiles following,

Vnguentum mundificatiuum.

℞ Olei Anethini, Olei Chamæmelini } ana. ℥.j.ß.
Olei Paralisis, Olei Petrolii } ana. ℥.i.
Misce.

Then I wrapp d all his neck, shoulder, arme, and hand with Emplastrum Diachalcitheos, & oxycroceum of each equall portions, by the which meanes those weake parts were recouered, and restored to their

former

former strength. Yée shall farther héere note in the time of his curing, I vsed also this approued mundificatiue with great benefit to the patient.

℞. Terebinthinæ ℥.ii.
Mellis Ros. ℥.i.
Succi Apii
Succi Plantaginis } ana.℥.ß.

Vnguentum mundificatiuum.

Let these séeth a little, and then adde thereunto
Farinæ Lupinorum
Farinæ Hordei } ana.ʒ.iii.
Sarcocollæ ʒ.i.
Croci.℈.i.
Misce.

Moreouer, I vsed Vnguentum Basilicon Maiestrale, and also Vnguentum Nicotian. and I laid outwardly vpon pledgets Emplastrum floris vnguentorum, and sometimes other plaisters and vnguents, as the cause required, & thus he was cured of the wound in his shoulder: as cõcerning the wound in the lower parts, I had no great trouble with it, but I perfected the cure with ordinary remedies, onely I am to giue you to vnderstand, that at the first I was troubled with a swelling, hardnes and inflammation in the testicles, which I remedied chiefly with this poultis.

℞. The crums of Rie bread, swéete butter, and the grounds of ale: but where ale is not to be had, then instéed therof I did take the grounds of strong béer: all these were boiled togither to the thicknes or forme of a poultis, and applied very warme: and so by these good meanes and helps he was cured. Thus I end this short obseruation, bicause I would be loth to be tedious, or to vse many superfluous words little auailable, and to no purpose &c.

A good poultis for swellings, hardnes, and inflammation of the testicles.

The cure of a Soldier that recieued a wound with a Musket bullet into the ioint, or bowing of his right arme, and also was pitifully burned with Gun pouder. Cap. 15.

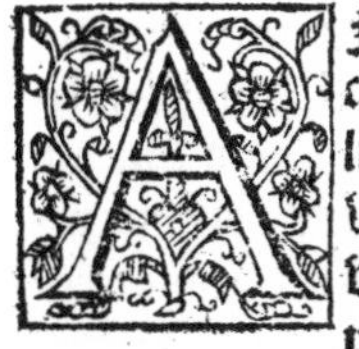

A Few yéeres agone in *Anno* 1586. I being in the Lowe countreis, there was brought vnto me to Arnam by lieutenant *Sing*, a soldier serning vnder Colonel *Morgan*, which was shot into the inside of his right arme in the very bowing of the ioint: presently vpon his hurt receiued, he began to linger and to stay after his companie.

Then there was one which he called his brother, perceiued him to be hurt, and not able to hold his péece, did presently venture himselfe and came vnto him to vnderstand the cause of his staying, and séeing him to be shot in, did vse all means possible to conuey him to the Surgeon to be drest: in fine, it happened by a misfortune, one of their flasks was fired, so that they were both greatly burned, especially this wounded mans hands, armes, and face, and in like sort his belly which tormented him very sore: for which cause I dressed him when he came to me, with Succum cæparum cum sale, ana. q.s. After I had vsed thrée or fower seuerall times this foresaid remedy, looke where I applied it, there neuer did rise any blisters, and the skin remained still one, but where I vsed it not, there were blisters store: to conclude, this cure of the burning was accomplished according as it is plainly set down in the beginning of this booke.

After I tooke a round blunt siluer probe, and gently put it into the wound, to trie the depth thereof, so by that meanes I found where the bullet laie in the very middle of his ioint, or bowing of his arme, and although the bullet was not far of, yet I could not possible so delate the wound with my instrument, that I might therewith take hold of the bullet, and the cause was the narownes and straightnes of the orifice or place where the bullet entred in, and therefore it was the more troublesome vnto me, doubting of the great distemperature, that otherwise might haue followed, but that was partly preuented by purging, and partly by his great losse of blood. And yée shall moreouer note, I was in more feare, in taking out of the shot, that I should do greater hurt by my incision, than was don at the beginning with the said bullet, bicause the sinewes, vaines and arteries were so néere at hand, whereby they could hardly be auoided: neuerthelesse, for that the bullet was great, I was constrained to inlarge the wound, that it might the more easilier come out: for although in fleshie places such bullets of Lead may rest without any great annoiance or danger vnto the bodie, yet being in a ioint or sinewie place, it may not there be suffred any time, if it be possible to be taken out. After I had inlarged that part by incision, then with much adoo, and great paines vnto the patient, I did take hold of the bullet with a Rostrum anatinum, yet do what I could with all curiositie, there followed (after my incision) a flure of blood, which mightily amazed the patient, and somwhat troubled me, but I staied it safely with my restrictiue powder. And although in some causes a flux of blood be not presently to be restrained, by reason the bléeding doth many times frée vs from inflammations, &c. yet may not excessiue and ouermuch bléeding be permitted, bicause the vitall spirits and naturall heat, do thereby waste and decaie, and greatly weaken the bodie. So after I had taken out the shot, I did put in my finger into the wound, to féele if there were any of the bone touched, but the first thing that offred it selfe to my finger was a péece of a rag or cloth, and bombace of his dublet which was carried in with the bullet, yet the bone was frée from any hurt that could be perceiued. So after the wound was fréed from all those annoiances, I presently did fill the wound with Olei Hyperici cum gummo, ℥.i. Olei ouorum ℥. ß. Then I applied outwardly vpon the same, (as I haue aboue said) to stay the bléeding, &c. And aboue the wound I laid this defensiue, to defend and kéepe backe fluxe of humors, for that he had a very full and plethoricke body.

A Defensiue.

℞. Olei Mirtini, Olei rosacei, ana. ℥. j. ß.
Olei Chamemeli ℥. j.
Boli Armeni ℥. iiij.
Omnium santalorum ana. ʒ. ij.
Sanguinis Draconis ℥. j.
Succi semperuini, Succi plantaginis, ana. ℥. ß.
Aceti rosarum ℥. ij.
Ceræ albæ q.s.
Misce.

First relent your oiles and iuices, and adde to your viniger, & boile all togither, then put in your waxe, & last your powders, after it is brought to a good body, reserue it to your vse. Thus with conuenient compressors and bindings, he rested very quietly for the space of thrée daies vndressed, by reason of the danger of his bléeding. And héere I thought it good to signifie vnto you, that in all my practise, I neuer found any great profit by the vse of Oleum catulorum, and such like remedies, in wounds of the ioints and sinewie places, but rather in those medicines, which are of a more strengthening and drying facultie: neither may Ægyptiacum in such sinewie places be vsed, though it be a medicine of ancient experience in the curing of Gun shot, by reason of his sharpe and biting qualitie, which I haue séene and knowen to bring many euill accidents, as paines, feuers, cramps, and conuulsions, &c. Therefore to preuent those dangers, I did with good aduice vse those remedies héere prescribed: then against the second dressing, which was the third day, I prepared new rowlers and bolsters, with cleane and swéete clothes for steuphs to foment the wound, with wine and Aqua vitæ: also I ordained in a readines Oleum rosarum & Albuminum ouorum q.s. mixed togither,

wherein

wherein I dipped thicke beds of towe, and warme applied them round about his ioint, which did greatly ease his paines, and tooke away the inflammation: and also I prepared this vnguent following, which I charged or spread vpon smal pledgets of lint, allwaies dipped in the foresaid oiles.

An Vnguent.

℞. Ceræ Citrinæ ℥.viij.
Resinæ ℥.iiij.
Terebinthinæ ℥.ij.
Thuris
Mastichis } ana.℥.j.
Olei Lumbricorum
Olei Nicotianæ } ana.℥.iij.
Misce.

Thus I continued this order of dressing thrée daies, and then I iniected into the wound with a syring this iniection following, ℞. Aquæ hordei lib.ij. Folior. Hyperici m.j. Vermium terrestrium ℥.iij. Sirr. Rosarum siccarum ℥.ij. Misce. These were boiled all togither till the third part was consumed: after I had two or thrée times togither well iniected the foresaid wound of his ioint, then very warme I ministred the foresaid oile of Hypericon and oile of egs, whereunto I added Mel Rosarum ℥.ß. and therein dipped pledgets of the vnguent before described, and ouer that, Emplastrum Nicotian. and very often the Gum plaister. And although there be many excellent plaisters seruing to this end and purpose, yet I suppose there are very few better: neuertheles, the best medicine that is, is no medicine, except it be in the hands of a skilfull man. And héere briefly to conclude this cure, ye shall note that all accidents were at the first mightily preuented with purging of his belly, sometimes with Cassia, and sometimes with clisters: bloodletting was omitted, for that he lost store at the first receiuing of his hurt. And so I finished this cure with other ordinarie vnguents and plaisters, in this booke by me truly and diligently published, &c.

The iniection

Nota.

The

The cure of a Smith, whose name was *William Hope*, belonging to the Tower of London, and one of hir Maiesties seruants, which vnfortunately receiued a shot through the thigh, with a bullet of Lead, out of an old Caliuer, which a long time had been charged, as heerafter shall bee said.

Cap. 16.

IN the yéere of our Lord 1584. I was sent for vnto the right honorable the Earle of Warwike: the cause was, that I would at his Lordships request take into my cure, the foresaid *William Hope* Smith, who was by his Honor preferred vnto the Quéenes Maiesties seruice, for his knowledge and skill in his art. The messenger that came vnto me was master *Richard Candish*, who signified vnto me his Lordships request, and how by ill hap, the poore man did shoote himselfe through his thigh with a bullet of Lead, out of an old rustie Caliuer, which had béene a long time charged, as it was supposed at the siege of Bullen, and so by some ouersight laid vp all that time, in the place or house of store within the Tower of London, and at a day of view taken of such old rustie péeces, this Caliuer was found charged with a bullet, and so deliuered vnto him, to haue the péece made seruiceable, and the bullet taken out: but as the patient confessed afterward, do what he could with all instruments and engins made for such purposes, it would not preuaile, but he was forced to put the bréech of the péece into the fire, and (not foreséeing the danger) did place, or rest the mouth of the saide péece, directly against the middle of his thigh, nothing suspecting that the péece would so suddenly haue blowen out the bullet: yet contrarie to his expectation, he shot himselfe through the thigh, whilest he did vse his one hand about the blowing of the bellowes, and his other hand in the framing and making of his fire. To procéede, there was brought vnto him a very expert and skilfull Chirurgion, that did take him in cure, but it was not his good hap to cure him, and for the space of thrée or fower yéeres he was constrained to go and stay himselfe with a staffe, by reason of the debilitie and weaknes of the part gréeued. After I had séene him and his gréefe, I found thrée great orifices outwardly, that were ve-

ry

ry neere togither and deepe, with much putrifaction inwardly. But ye shall note, the first indication of curing was performed by Doctor *Randall*, for the purging and euacuating of those humors abounding. The next day following, he was let blood ten or twelue ounces, being very foule blood, and of an ill colour: his meats were easie of digestion, and of good nourishment, by reason he had a bad stomacke to his meate. The second scope of curing was performed after this maner, I laid aboue the wound, and so round about the compasse of his greefe, that defensiue which is published in the ninth chapter of this booke, that done, I did vse the causticke stone, vpon the vttermost part of his greefe, where by due application thereof, done with my owne hand, I brought all the three orifices into one, in lesse than a quarter of an houre: by this inlargement the greefe was of a sufficient wideneсse, after the eschars were remoued, then I found the circuits or solution of vnitie great, and the corrupt flesh abounding with hils and banks very proudly growne, the humors that continually flowed, were pale, glutinous, and of a bad sauor: neuertheles, by little and little, I subdued all the superfluous and spungeous flesh, with these medicines, which are of a sharpe and biting qualitie, some gentler, as Mercurij præcipitati, and some stronger, as that powder which is published in the third Chapter of this booke: and somtimes I vsed this mundificatiue following, so that by these meanes, of an old vlcer was made a fresh wound,

A. pare.

℞. Pulueris aluminis rochæ
Viridis æris
Vitrioli Romani
Mellis rosati } ana. ℥. ii.
Aceti boni q. s.

Bulliant omnia simul secundum artem, & fiat medicamentum ad formam mellis.

Also I did oftentimes iniect with a syring into the bottom of his greefe, this foresaid ointment with wine and Aqua vitæ, and somtimes the ointment alone warmed vpon dossels and pledgets of lint, and for that I was vnacquainted with the nature and disposition of his body, by reason of the ill habite thereof, so that after the greefe was well mundified and clensed, and his body prepared as aforesaid, in the end I did giue him that to drinke, called Potus Antiochiæ, and also I did iniect of the same drinke into the wound without addition, after I applied Vnguentum incarnatiuum, and somtimes Vnguentum basilicon vpon pledgets dipped in the said drinke being warmed, and the gum plaister all ouer: by this meanes his greefe did yeelde perfect white digestiue matter, & the holownes and lost substance of flesh was againe restored

by

by the helpe of these medicines and the benefit of nature, notwithstanstanding in the end of the cure, it made some stay in the cicutrizing or sealing vp, which I performed with that sparadrop plaister, published in the foure and twentith chapter of this booke, and is of my M. *Kebles* description, and thus he was perfectly healed, and so remaineth vnto this day.

The cure of a Seruingman, which was shot into the leg with a sheafe arrow, and the head sticking in the bone. Cap. 17.

A Few yeeres past, at a great mustering and training vp of soldiers at Mile-end greene, neer London: Amongst those bands of trained men, there was appointed a certaine number of Archers: who after they had marched a long time, in the end the bowe men were diuided from the pikemen and shot, onely to trie and exercise their bowes: it chanced in their shooting at a marke, about six or seauen score off, by misfortune one of their arrowes did hit a gentlemans seruant called master *Withipole*, into the outside of his left leg, so that the shaft was firmly fixed in the bone, yet being a good way off beyond the marke, when he receiued his hurt. There was at that time one in the field which professed Surgery, and proffered to dresse the wound, presently in the place where the patient was hurt: he being in great pains, was glad of any helpe, and so permitted the fellow to dresse him, who forthwith did attempt to take out the arrow, nothing regarding the renting or tearing of the muscles, but ouer hastily, and vnaduisedly, did pull out the shaft, and left the arrow head fast fastened in the bone, being a barbed head, as are commonly all our English sheafe arrowes. After willingly he would haue excused the matter, and seemed to say, that the head was ill glued or fastened to the arrow, and so he dressed the patient, to his freendes great disliking: for that the patient was immediately troubled and molested with a hot distemperature, much paines, and vnmeasurable swellings, which induced a feuer, and his stomack cleane taken from his meate. Then it was the will and pleasure of one master *Spinolo*, in Fanchurch streete where I did dwell to send for me, and there I found the Surgeon, but his patient being in extreme paines: wherefore in my presence, for that they would be rid of this fellow, they said they were greatly agreeued with him, and told him he had stained his practise, in preseruing and dressing the patient so ill, and that his abuse was great and deserued punishment. Then he went about to bleare their eies with a little beggerly eloquence, the which he had learned amongst a sort of trecherous runnagates, counterfet land lopars, Sophisticall mounty-banks, cosoning quacksaluers, and such like false iugling deceiuers, with their paradoxicall innouations, whose natiue soile is to them a wilde cat, and who abuse all good Arts, wheresoeuer they come or abide. But to omit circumstances, I say he vanished away in darknes, as may appeare in my former books, where I haue more at large spoken of him and other the like abusers, whose bloddy hands without knowledge, do hazard the liues of many.

Nota.

1 Such emptie barrels sound farre,
Which do little good in peace or warre:
It is a world to vnderstand,
How such do florish in this land.

2 Long haue I mused at the same,
Till I perused stories old:
Where I did finde men of much fame,
Greatly dislike such persons bold.

3 Wherefore I leaue them to their wils,
That list to like these kinde of men:
And when they haue approoued their skils,
They may the better iudge of them.

4 Now in the end I thus conclude,
They were none of the sons of Art:
But men vnskilfull grosse and rude,
Euen as the blinde man casts his dart.

After he was gone, I remoued all things from the patients leg, and I did put downe a probe into the bottom of the wound, where manifestly I did feele the head fixed in the bone, and by reason the orifice of the wound was so straight & swolne, that I could not dilate any instrument

ment sufficiently to apprehend and take hold of the arrow head, therfore I was driuen to make reasonable large incision downe to the bottome, and then did put into the place of my incision Adilatorium to open the wound, and so presently tooke hold of the arrow head with a Rostrum gruinum, and then moued it by little & little, so very gently with safety I tooke out the arrow head, and after I put my finger into the wound, to feele if there were any rough fragments or shiuers of the bone, but I found none at all: then after I suffered him to bleed a reasonable quantity, for that he bled but very litle when he receiued his hurt: after I preserued the wound with Oleum Aparisij very hot, and laid round about the parts this defensatiue.

A defensiue.

℞. Diachalcitheos
Olei papaueris
Olei rosarum rubarum
Aceti ros. } ana. q. s.
Misce.

And I staied in the end his bleeding with my restrictiue powder, and also I ordained this cooling medicine, which did greatly helpe to qualifie his hot distemperature, and did mitigate his paines, and staied the flux of humors,

A cooling Vnguent.

℞. Vnguenti nutriti
Vnguenti rosarum } ana. ℥. iiii.
Succi plantaginis
& Solani } ana. q. s.
Misceantur in mortario plumbeo, &c.

Then I ministred round about the swelling that Cataplasma, which is published in the fift Chapter of this booke. After that with conuenient rowlings, such as were rather for commodity than for fashion sake, I very easily rowled it vp, & so finished this first dressing. The next day early in the morning he was new drest againe, for that he was not free from his feuer, though his pains were somwhat appeased, and his swellings well vanished away. Then after his dressing he was let blood on the liuer vaine, by the counsell of a Physition and the next day he receiued a clister with order of diet prescribed: for locall remedies I followed mine owne experience, with poultises defensatiues and cooling ointments, as afore I haue said: and after as occasion was offered, I vsed Emplastrum cum gummis, & Vnguentum de peto, or Nicotion with Oleum Aparisij, and vsually steuphs of wine: the rest of his curing was like the cure of other greene wounds, which I haue particularly specified in many parts of this booke &c.

The cure of a man, which receiued a notable wound in his head with great fracture of the skull : and did moreouer fracture the bone of his thigh called *Os femoris*, by a fall out of a gallery in the Beare garden, at that time when all the gallery there did fall downe, and killed and hurt many. Cap. 18.

I Haue thought it good afore I enter into this briefe note or obseruation, first to signifie vnto the yong practisers of Chirurgery: that al such great wounds in the head, with fracture of the skull, are holden generally of the best writers and practisers, to be most perilous and dangerous: the bone being compressed vpon Dura mater. For the which cause, at the very beginning of this cure, I did cut and shaue away the haire round about the wound, then with my fingers I made further probation into the wound, and there I did manifestly feele a notable fracture or breach in the skull on the left side of his head, vpon the bone called Os petrosum, which (as I said) was depressed vpon the pannicle Dura mater, and for that the fracture of the skull was greater in length, than the wound in the flesh, for that cause without detracting of time I made incision, and so followed the fracture vntill all the rift or crackt bone was wholy discouered. When I did see and behold the full length of the fracture or breach in the skull, & had made a sufficient dilatation, and raised vp the flesh: for that cause I could not at that present time proceed any further, by reason of the great flux of blood: and moreouer, for that he lost much blood before he was brought to his lodging: all which being considered, I filled the wound with pledgets and runlets made of lint and very fine towe, wet in the whites of egs mixed with *Galen* his pouder: then with good bolstring and rowling he thus remained vntill the next day, and then likewise hauing a present regard vnto the preseruation of the fracture of his thigh, the maner and order thereof heereafter shall be declared. But before I enter any further into this discourse, I thought it good heere to note, that this patient was a man of some account, & for that cause his master was very desirous to vnderstād of me what danger he was in, bicause he would acquaint other of his friends in the countrey therewith. Then I considered I was to speake with men of worship and good calling, vnto whom I deliuered mine opinion: but first calling to remembrance some part of the wise sayings of *Guido*, *Tagaltius* and others, whose counsell in this case ought of vs to be reuerenced

reuerenced and imbraced.

When thou art called (say they) before a magistrate or head officer, so " that thou art required to deliuer thine opinion, sentence, and iudgement " vpon the person wounded, & to prognosticate as much as art requireth, it " behoueth thée, diligently & effectually to marke the wound or wounds, if " there be many & thou shalt truly cal the same wound or wounds by their " expresse & proper names, togither with the place woũded. Then after it " behoueth thée to consider with thy selfe the cause of thy coniecture, & the " reason of thy sentence and iudgement by thée deliuered wisely and pru- " dently, least thou faile in thy iudgement, and shew thy selfe to be either " ignorant or els deceiued. So hauing these precepts in my memory, I told them, he was not without great danger, partly by reason the braine was sore shaken with the fall, and partly for that the bone was broken and depressed vpon Dura mater, which were the causes that did hinder his spéeches, and that could not be remedied at the first dressing, by reason of the great flux of blood: Howbeit I did hope of some amendment, after I had pearced the skull with the Trepan. Other talke I had as touching the ill signes of his vomiting, the greatnes of his wound, with the fracture of his skull and thigh, whereof I will speake more largely in discourse of his curing. And for that I would be very wary and circumspect, I caused them to hang all his chamber with Carpets and Couerlids, and made it very darke, without light or aire but onely by a candle, bicause in this case, the aire is very hurtfull. Which done, at the second preseruation, after I had vnrowled his head, and taken out of the wound, all things that were administred for the restraining of the flure of blood. And for that a vent was to be made with all expedition, for the matter and congealed blood to come forth, therefore I caused a strong man stedfastly to hold and stay his head with his hands, and hauing stopped his eares with wooll, I then did set on the Trepan, and so orderly pearsed the skull through in two places: then with an instrument called a Leuator, I raised vp the depressed bone: which being done, immediately his spéech amended. And there was found vpon Dura mater, a good quantitie of congealed blood, which was remoued with fomentations of wine, Aqua vitæ, and other remedies, as héereafter shall be declared. It is further to be noted, that there did manifestly appéer vpon Dura mater a certaine blacknes: for which cause I did put betwéen the Dura mater and the skull, a péece of fine Lawne, in the stead of Sindan that *Vigo* commendeth, dipped in Mel rosarum, and Aqua vitæ ana. q.s. And with lint wet in the same I filled vp the wound: and at other times I vsed Vnguentum Caprifolij, which I found described in master *Gales* second booke of his Antidotarie, and likewise it is extant in *Wecker*, and in diuers

other

other good authors.

Vnguentum Caprifolij. Wecker.

℞. Terebinthinæ, Resinæ pini, Ceræ nouæ ana. ℥.iiij.
Olei rosati ℥.viij.
Mastichis, Thuris ana. ℥.j.
Gummi Elemni ℥.ij.
Caprifolij, Betonicæ ana. ℥.iij.
Vini optimi lib.x.

These herbs being stamped, let them stand infused in the wine fower and twenty howers, then adde to them all the other parcels except the Gums, Frankincense, and Masticke: boile these on a cleere fire vntill halfe the wine be consumed, and that it begin to wax greene, then strain it, and let it coole: then boile it againe, till all the wine be wasted, then straine it: and lastly adde to the Masticke and Thuris made in very fine powder: put it after in a cold place, and reserue it to your vse. After (as I said) I had preserued the wound with these remedies, then I applied heerewithall, a plaister of Betonie, and I annointed his head round about the wound Cum oleo rosarum, and ouer all this a good bed or cap of towe, and then with bolstering and rowling, I finished this dressing, &c.

Emplastrum Betonicæ.

℞. Gummi Elemni ℥.iiij.
Resinæ ℥.viij.
Ceræ ℥.vj.
Gummi Ammoniaci ℥.iiij.
Terebinthinæ ℥.vj.
Succi Betonicæ ℥.x.
Misce, & fiat emplastrum.

I was constrained, contrarie vnto the first description of this plaister, to double the quantities of all the simples, bicause I did vse very much of it: and thus I continued with this maner of dressing, vntill all the blacknes was taken away from the Dura mater, by the vse of the foresaid hony of roses. But if the blacknes should not haue gone away, notwithstanding the vse of hony of roses, as I haue often seene, then the cure is to be feared, and small hope of health to be looked for. And heere I say againe, this wounded man was in the more danger, for that he receiued his hurt very neere vnto the full of the moone, whereby this euill followed, that Dura mater did rise and thrust it selfe, out of those places of the skull, that I did perforate or pearce with the Trepan, the which

which I did safely bring downe againe with this decoction or fomentation,

A Decoction.

R. Fol. Ros.
Chamæmeli
Meliloti
Betonicæ } ana. m. j.
Aquæ vitæ q. s.

These were well boiled togither in faire water, and last of all was added the Aqua vitæ, and herewith I did well bathe and foment the place, and then applied upon Dura mater, this remedie following, with a fine peece of lawne, which was orderly conueied under Cranium, or the skull, to defend the pannicle from being hurt with the sharpe edge of the bone,

R. Olei rosarum
Mellis rosarum } ana. ℥. j.
Aquæ vitæ ℥. ß.
Misce.

And somtimes also I used for that purpose Oleum Vitellorum ouorum: and further ye shall note, that upon the forenamed peece of lawne, I placed a small peece of a spunge steeped in the decoction, and so by this meanes Dura mater was safely brought downe againe, which to do in some bodies is wonderfull hard and difficult, therefore it doth require great care, diligence, and skill. And as touching the scaling of the fractured bones, it was safely done in a reasonable time and space, partly with the use of Oleum rosarum & Aqua vitæ, and partly with Aqua vitæ & Vitriol. albi ana. q. s. But when I applied the Aqua vitæ and Vitriol. I did first defend the fleshie parts with dry lint, &c. which otherwise would haue caused very great paines and griefe: neither is it meete that such great wounds should be disquieted with any sharpe or biting medicines, which often do greatly hinder the perfection and course of the cure: for that cause it is thought most profitable to use chiefly Puluis cephalicus, as a very apt and conuenient remedie, for scaling of bones of the head. And with these foresaid medicines I continued, untill there was perfect flesh upon Dura mater: and the fractured bones being losed, and borne up so in place of these bones, nature ordained and supplied a good and perfect Callus. And by this method and maner of curing, in the end he was well and perfectly healed of this wound in the head. Also ye shall further understand, that in the course of his curing, we were compelled to use good diet, purging and bleeding, which was performed by the aduice and counsell of a Physition. Now heere I will also very briefly speake of the fracture of the bone of his thigh: First I did endeuour my

selfe

selfe for the right placing of this fractured member, which was broken tranuerse or crossewise: it is againe to be further noted, that of fractures when they happen in bodies of an euill disposition and temperature, they ostentimes resist cure, and are long or euer they be made whole. This patient was a man of a yong and lusty body, and so of a very good constitution, then after I say, he was brought to his bed, and orderly laid vpon his backe: which being done, I made two decent towels, and fastened each towell, one aboue the fracture, and the other below it: then I caused two strong men to apprehend and take hold of each towell, and I placed my selfe very neere vnto the fracture: then all things being readie, I caused them to extend or stretch out the member very strongly, which being sufficiently performed, I did eleuate or lift vp that part of the bone which was depressed, and againe, I did also presse downe the other part of the fractured bone which was borne vp, and being rightly reduced, and restored againe, as neere as I could to natures former vnion, I did curiously keepe close togither the parts before disseuered: and then caused the two men, which extended the member, by little and little to release their hands, whereby the patient found himselfe greatly eased. After this done, I did take linnen clothes so large, as did not onely comprehend the fracture, but also couered ouer some of the whole and sound parts, the which cloth I did wet in water and viniger, and being well wrung out, I did spread vpon it this remedie heere described,

Keble.

℞. Albuminis ouorum
Olei rosarum
Boli Armeniaci
Farinæ volatilis } ana. q. s.

Many excellent men do also vse to wet the said cloth in Albuminis ouorum, & Olei rosarum, ana.q.s. being first well beaten togither: and after being reasonably compressed out againe, do apply it to the part afflicted, and I my selfe haue approued it most certaine true. But I did vse the aboue rehearsed remedies, with good successe as I haue declared, and therwith compassed the member three or fower times, then with decent rowlers made of soft linnen cloth, which also were wet in water and viniger called Posca. I did begin my ligature or rowling directly vpon the fracture, and so rowled it vpwards, twise or thrise togither, and after rowled it downwards: and in like maner ascending vpwards againe aboue the fracture. Thus after the same order as before, I did again rowle it with another rowler of the same bredth and length, that is to say, two yards long and fower fingers broad, then according vnto *Horatius Morus* direction, and others who say: your maner of rowling must

must neither be too straight, neither yet too loose: for by ouer loose binding the bones they may be moued, & by too straight & ouer hard girding doth hinder the distribution of nourishment into the part, & so letteth the ingendring or breeding of the sodring humor, wherwith the bones are vnited & knit, which is said to be made of good nourishmēt inclining to grosnes. Now to come vnto the maner & order of the placing of the splints, which were orderly set and placed vpon the said rowlers, which splints were made of light willow wood, being very plaine and smooth, and blunt and round at both the ends, well wrapped about, and also bolstered with towe, which I placed then, as I said, the bredth of a finger betweene euery splint, and somtimes farther off or neerer, as the cause required: then with good strong tape I did very gently binde them well togither: which being done, I laid or placed the member as seemely and decently as possibly might be, in a double linnen towel rouled vp at both ends, with a good quantitie of long rushes, such as our Chandlers vse to put into their watching candles: and I did make thereof as it were a bed to lay or place the fractured member in, so that he could by no means any way moue his fractured leg: but safely and quietly he rested, as though it had been laid into that famous instrument called Glossocominum The true order and right vse therof, was first showen and made plaine vnto me, and diuers other Chirurgions, by master Doctor *Foster*, a most learned gentleman, Reader of the Chirurgery lecture in the Physitions college in London. To proceede, after I had safely laid in his leg as aforesaid, then he rested reasonably quiet for the space of fourteene daies, and then suddenly without any reasonable cause knowne, there did begin to rise a very painful itch, and withal an inflammation: then I followed the direction of *Wecker*, and fomented the member with warme water, to this end and purpose, that the humors which were compact and inclosed, might the more easily euaporate and breath out: which done, I annointed the member round about with Vnguentum populeon compositum, & Vnguentum album camphoratum, ana. q. s. Then I vsed also this plaister,

℞. Emplastri Diachalcitheos ℥. viii.
Olei mirtillorum ℥. i. ß.
Succi granatorum ℥. i.
Albumin. ouorum numero ii.
Misce.

After I did rowle vp the member againe in the same maner and order as is before declared. And thus by the vse of these remedies, his itch and inflammation was remoued & taken away without further trouble, and so in a reasonable time he was made whole of the fracture of his thigh, and for that it stood me vpon to haue regard and great care vnto this agreeued patient, I did diuers times call with me to visit him M. *Banister*, whose counsell herein was vnto me very profitable. To conclude, after I had fully ended the cure of my patient, then both he and his freends, seemed to be discontented with me, for that the fractured member was somwhat shorter than his other leg: I told them againe, it was not to be helped in him: yet much may be done in yong people, which in aged persons did not so luckily fall out, as we wish & looke for: so they departed from me, being not well pleased for the shortnes of his leg, and I much more discontented for their base minded paiment for the healing of so great and dangerous a cure.

An obseruation of the cure of a fractured thigh, don vpon a yoong boy of ten yeeres of age.

And here calling to minde a few yeeres past, a yong boy being about the age of ten yeeres, whose name is called *Martin Aude*, who did commonly resort vnto a brewers house in Bishops gate streete, where he also did dwell: in the same brewhouse there was a horse mill, that did grinde the brewers malt, and there this boie with other such like youths, resorted to play, and vnaduisedly running about the mill, by mishap the mill did catch holt of his cote, and so did pull or draw him to the mill, in such sort, that the mil stone did run ouer his thigh, and fractured Os femoris in diuers peeces, then by reason of his noise and crying, the felow that did leade the horse, very suddenly staied the mill, otherwise all his whole body had been drawn into the mill, and so crushed and broken in peeces. Then I was sent for, and master *George Baker*, one of hir Maiesties Chirurgions, whose soundnes in practise is answerable to his calling. I might hereunto annexe to his great commendations, his compendious works of Surgerie, by him published in the English tong, for the helpe and comfort of many of hir Maiesties good subiects. But to returne, I say we being both togither, presently placed againe the fractured bones, and also applied thereto meete and conuenient remedies, and so in a reasonable time, with great and diligence, we made him perfect whole and sound of that leg without lamenesse, or any other imperfection whatsoeuer, and he liueth at this day, &c.

An obseruation for the cure of a master of a Hoy, that had both his legs fractured and broken into many peeces, with an iron bullet, shot out of a great basse or harquebusse of crocke at the sea, by a Pirot or sea rouer.

Cap. 19.

FRéendly Reader, I haue in the chapter going before, manifested vnto you, and spoken of two great and dangerous cures of fractured bones of the thigh, which by the helpe and singular goodnes of God were accomplished, as you haue heard declared. Now it remaineth that here in this chapter also I make a bréefe rehersal of a certaine master of a Hoy, which a few yéeres past, sailing on the seas, was chased by a Pirot or sea rouer, who being in a ship of war, shot at him with a great basse or harquebusse of crock, and did hit or strike the said master of the Hoy, with an iron bullet through both the smals of his legs, and fractured all the bones asunder, and also did rend and teare the muscles, tendons, nerues, vaines and arteries, and so made two notable great wounds in both his legs. By reason héerof, and also of his being long vndrest, there followed after diuers euill symtomes, as a feuer, troublesome shiuerings, vehement paines, inflammations, tumors, and likewise strange fluxes of blood, which procéeded by reason of the magnitude, and greatnes of the wound: but moreouer, that which was more preiudiciall and cloied vs very greatly, was a Gangræna. Now héere you shall vnderstand, I was sent for vnto this great and dangerous cure, and also master *Crowe*, and master *Wood*, Chirurgeons of London, being men of long experience: the reason was, for that this worke was greater than it had béene possible for one man to performe: and then the patient being aboord his Hoy some ten or twelue miles from London néere vnto the great breach, and could not come vp by reason the wind and tide was against him, then at the request of his friends we all thrée went downe the riuer to him. And when we came aboord his Hoy, we found him lying vpō the hatchets néer vnto the helme where he receiued his wounds, then presently we laid open all the gréeued parts, and finding the worke so great, that hardly could any of our helpes haue béene mist, therefore first of al we made ready to dres him such remedies as we had about vs, and as the time and place would serue: which don, we did with as much lenity and ease as possible we could, take away much stinking coagulat and clottered blood: then we remoued certaine of the loose shiuers and péeces of fractured bones, that done, we made a straight and easie extention as it was possible for vs to do it, for feare of wresting or shaking of the fractured members, holding our hands very stedfastly aboue and belowe the fractures, least the bones should haue béen remoued out of their places: so we drest them according to art, & after rowled them vp, leauing cõuenient places for vs to dresse the wounds at, and a méete way for nature to vnburthen hir selfe of corruptions: which don, we applied thereon our splints and other necessary supportings, as it is declared in the last Chapter going before, after we laid both his legs from the féete vnto the groin as straight as possibly might be, & after bound them vp with conuenient ligatures, then he was laid in a bote and brought vp with vs to London, and placed in a very good lodging, where we drest him again more orderly with fomentations, and other conuenient remedies, according to the old beaten way and doctrine of *Vigo*, and other ancient fathers, whose authorities confirmed our experience in this cure. Last of all I must néeds say, truly, it was a long time after or euer the bones of his legs were perfectly cõfirmed with a callow, and so able to go without paine, yet in the end God gaue vs a fortunate successe, and he was cured by vs, but with a callow somwhat greater, than willingly we would it should haue béen, and some imperfection in the straightnes of his legs, notwithstanding all our faithfull care & diligence to the contrary, yet he liueth at this day and goeth strongly vpon both his legs, without staffe or stay to support himselfe by &c.

The cure of a Mariner, which had two of his ribs fractured and broken, with the violent blow of a Capisten barre, in one of hir Maisties ships called the Aide, which brused him very sore: at the same present time he was throwen downe vpon the cariage of a great peece of ordinance, which brused him againe in other parts of his body. Cap. 20.

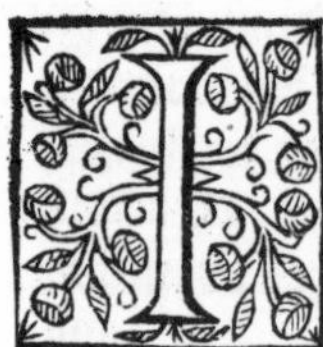

Think it good, without any longer discourse, so briefly as I can, héere to publish and plainly to expresse the truth of my practise in this cure, & with al faithfulnes, industry, and diligence, to procéede vnto the rest, as I haue said. It happened at that time, when the Emperours daughter passed

passed the narrow seas, to marry with *Philip* king of Spaine. I seruing then in one of hir Maiesties ships called the Aide, it chanced that a great tempest and winde did rise, so that the billowes and surging waues of the sea went very lofty and high, we riding then at our anchor néere the French coast, and the Marriners being greatly busied about the winding vp of their cables and anchors: it happened by reason of the storme and tempest, and by some negligence and ouersight, vpon a sudden the Capisten turned about with great force and violence, and did bruse and hurt diuers, specially the boteswaines seruant, whose name was called *Ralfe Condall*, which had two of his ribs fractured and broken by the force of the said blowe of the Capisten barre, and therewith throwne downe vpon the carriage of a great péece of ordinance, which brused him againe in other places of his body: so the patient did lie as a dead man void of sence and vnderstanding, neither did he remember or know whether he had béene drest or no. But after he was again reuiued, there followed perilous accidents, as a Pleurisie, spitting of blood, & gret dolor and pains, which (as *Guido* declareth) are very dangerous, and the rather for that one of his ribs was in such sort fractured, that a little fragment or small péece of the rib, did separate it selfe without all hold vnto any part of the rib, which continually without ceasing still tormented and vexed the patient, with vehement prickings vpon the panicle that couereth the ribs, neither could I bring him to any ease, vntill I did make incision directly vpō the fracture, according vnto the length of the rib, and so downe vnto the bone: and there I did take out that shiuer or spell of the bone, which was in bignes, thicknes, and length like vnto a barly corne, sharpe at both ends like vnto the point of a néedle. Then after I had made the incision, and taken out the small péece of the bone, I applied into the said wound Oleum hyperici cum gummo, and then vpon the same, for the more spéedy vniting and kniting of the fractured ribs togither, this remedy following,

℞. Olei Rosarum
Albuminis ouorum
Boli Armoniaci
Farinæ volutilis } ana.q.s.

The which I spread vpon a double linnen cloth being first wet in water and viniger, & strongly wrong out again. But you shall vnderstand for that there was not at that time any Physition in the Nauie to aide and asist me in this cure, therefore I gaue him my selfe to drinke this potion following, which wrought after this maner: for within one hower after, he did cast mightily, not onely the most part of his drinke, but also a good quantity of congealed or clotted blood withal, neuertheles at night I

gaue

gaue him the same drinke againe, and so continued for the space of thrée daies, al which time he did neuer offer to cast vp any thing, but onely by spitting at his mouth, and so he did auoid much brused blood, and this is the foresaid drinke,

A drink very good for bruses inwardly.

℞. Vini maluatici ℥.iiij.
Olei Oliuarum dul. ℥.j.
Spermatis ceti gra. xii.
Misce.

Now héere it is also to be noted, that after the said péece of the bone of his rib was taken out, he neuer greatly complained of any paines in that part, but he was further troubled with a cough which he had taken before he receiued his hurt, for that cause and for the more spéedy cure of his fractured ribs, I did giue him to drinke for the space of ten daies, morning and euening, this drinke following,

Master Welliseds drinke, Surgeon of Douer.

℞. Aquæ consolidæ maioris & } ana. ℥.ij.
Aquæ Osmundæ regalis }
Vini albi ℥.iiij.
Mellis comm. ℥.iij.
Succi Liqueritiæ ʒ.j.
Theriacæ opt. q.s.
Misce.

This drinke did profit the patient greatly, and was first giuen vnto me for a singular secret, by one master *Wellised* Chirurgion, then dwelling at Douer, néere vnto the sea coast, with whom I had conference about this cure. And héerewithall ye shall note, that I gaue him likewise a very gentle purge onely to cleanse the belly, and also I did let him blood: all which were great helpes for the perfection of this cure. And thus orderly from time to time I procéeded. After the like maner I vsed locall remedies, as is before said, and also héerafter following, with méete and conuenient bolstering and rowling: and euery fift day he was new drest by reason of the wound, and at the tenth daies end the wound was perfectly healed. The tenth day being expired, I changed my course of dressing, and vsed this maner and order following,

℞. Emplastrum Diachalcitheos } ana. ℥.iiij.
Emplastrum Deminio }
Olei Rosarum & } ana. ℥.j.
Olei Mirtillorum }
Misce.

These plaisters thus incorporated did confirme and strengthen the foresaid broken ribs, and I annointed him also in other parts of his bodie where he was sore brused, with these oiles,

℞. Olei

℞. Olei Rosarum & } ana.℥.j.
Olei Chamæmeli }
Olei spermatis ceti ℥.ß.
Misce.

And many times likewise I vsed Vnguentum Dialtheæ, Oleum laurinum, & Vnguentum Vulpinum, and moreouer I resolued all the contused & brused blood, which was inclosed vnder the skin, with the aforesaid oiles, and also with application of these plaisters following,

℞. Emplastri de Mucilagibus }
Emplastri de Meliloto } ana.℥.ij.
Emplastri de flore vnguentorum }
Olei Chamæmeli } ana.ʒ.vj.
Olei Rosarum }
Misce.

At the fifteene daies end I opened the wound againe, where I found it as I said before, perfectly healed, and also the fractured ribs very apparently to haue receiued consolidation: & thus I end this short discourse, omitting to speake of the order of his diet, which was sparing ynough in the highest degree.

The cure of a certaine man, that was thrust through his body with a sword, which did enter first vnder the cartilage or gristle, called of the Anatomists *Mucronata Cartilago* and the point of the sword passed through his body and so out at his backe, in such maner that he which wounded the man did run his way, and did leaue the sword sticking in his bodie: so the wounded man did with his owne hands pull out the sword, whom after I cured as shall be heere declared. Cap.21.

A Speciall note or obseruation of a certaine dangerous and desperate cure in my simple iudgement, worthy of admiration, of a certaine traueller into the coasts of India, and other far countries, being a very valiant and strong person: who (as I said) receiued a wound through his body, which entred in vnder Mucronata Cartilago, but by the wonderfull worke of God the sword escaped the liuer, the

the stomacke, and the intestines or guts: for there were no manifest signes of any of those parts to be offended and hurt, neither any euill accidents happened, during all the time of this cure, but onely the grudging of a feuer, which followeth such wounds, as the shadow doth the body: and that was shortly preuented by bleeding, and loosing of the belly with soluble clisters. Presently vpon his hurt receiued, I was called vnto this cure, and likewise one master Doctor *Wotton*: but to speake the truth, after I did behold the maner of his hurt, and seeing the weapon so imbrued with blood, I did in my mind greatly lament his mishap, and tolde those that were in presence, that I doubted much there was no hope of cure in him, but that death would very shortly follow, and so I was vnwilling to dresse him, supposing he would die vnder my hand. Then the wounded patient desired me (as I loued a man) that I would dresse him, and take him in cure: for (said he) my hart is good, although my wound be great. Then I called to my remembrance the learned counsell of *Celsus*, who willeth vs in no wise to meddle with him that cannot be preserued, nor to deale with him that is slaine alreadie: yet to counteruaile this, I read in other good authors, that we ought in conscience to attempt all that may possible be done, either by art or reason for the safetie of the patient: but first warily to foretell what danger the patient is in, before ye shall either make or meddle with him, that you may defend your selues from the slander of euill speakers. For say these excellent men, many by a woonderfull and miraculous maner do escape death and are cured. Therefore as I haue said in the Chapters going before, if we shall leaue the wounded man destitute of all aide and helpe, and so he die, we shall worthily be called and esteemed wicked, and without all charitie and humanitie. But (friendly reader) often times it so falleth out, that many worthy and skilfull Artists, are most fearfull, and very vnwilling to enterprise and attempt any such great and dangerous cures, partly by reason of the slanders of backbiters, and others of the like rude sort of euill speakers: for if it so fall out at any time, that some one disordered or vnfortunate patient die, or chaunce to escape vncured, by reason of the greatnes of the griefe or disease, then a man shall be condemned without mercie, notwithstanding all honest endeuours truly performed, neuer once considering that we cannot enter into Gods diuine prouidence, to foretell, know, and vnderstand, whether it be his good will and pleasure, to grant health and recouerie vnto the sicke or wounded patient or not. Howbeit this I know assuredly, a man shall get more discredit and infamous reports by such bad patients, than euer they got credit by all the famous cures they haue done all the daies of their liues. But I suppose there is no Surgeon that is a true

Christian,

Christian, will willingly and of set purpose, as some haue said, do that which redoundeth to his patients hurt and ouerthrow, which cannot be but to his owne shame and vtter vndoing in this world, besides the high displeasure of almightie God in the world to come. I hope and am fully perswaded, it will be too hard for any of those slanderers to search out, & worse to find any such foul & odious abuses to raign & be amongst vs. But to returne, I say, after much intreating, I enterprised this cure as followeth: I did first take two short tents artificially made, the one for the fore part of his breast, and the other for behinde his backe: vpon the which tents I applied *Galen* his powder, mixed with hares haires, and the whites of egs, and so put them into the wound: and vpon the said tents outwardly certaine pledgets, being also spred with the foresaide restrictiue. Moreouer, the wound was defended both before and behind, with very good defensiues, and also artificiall bolstering and rowling: he so rested vntill the third day, for feare of the bleeding. In the meane space, the foresaid Doctor of Physicke with others agreed, forthwith to giue the patient some excellent wound drinke: the Doctor consented that we should administer such as by our owne experience and practise, we had well approued. Then I told him of the singular vertues, which I had heard and seene of a certaine wound drinke, called Potus Antiochiæ, which was first put in practise in London, by a very skilfull Chirurgion called Master *Archenboll.* The strange cures which the said drinke hath done, are wonderfull to heare, and this wounded man was cured chiefly with this drinke of Antioch. The maner and order of ministring and making of it, is as followeth,

Potus Antiochiæ.

℞. Bugulæ
Fragariæ
Consolidæ mediæ
Consolidæ minoris
Consolidæ maioris
Raphani rusticani
Rubi
Vrticæ fœmineæ
Osmundæ
Canabis
Saniculæ
Crasulæ
Tanaceti
Anagallidis masculi
Auriculæ muris
Violarum purpurearum } ana. m. i.

Garyophyllatæ cum radicibus & foliis m. v.
Geranii Cretici m. v.
Betonicæ cum radicibus, & foliis m. v.
Pedis columbini cum radicibus, & foliis, m. iii.

Rubiæ tinctorum of the roots, the third part in waight of al the herbs, before rehearsed, first wash all the herbes cleane, then after stampe them in a stone morter, which done, put them all in a new earthen pot well nealed, and put thereto also a gallon of good white wine: then set them on an easie fire of coles, & let thē boile very gently till the one halfe be consumed, then straine them into a faire cleane vessell, & ad to them, of the best and purest clarified honie one gallon, so that there be of ech an equall quantitie: then boile them togither, as it is said in the ancient copie, the time and space yée may say the Psalme of Mercie: and it must alwaies be giuen blood warme, one spoonfull at a time (first and last) morning and euening, in well water, thrée spoonfuls at a time, being sodden and kept vpon purpose: and I know that this drinke hath béen ministred after it was ten yéeres old. I say I did by fréndship get (of one master *Bedon* Chirurgeon) so much of this drinke, that chéefly cured this wounded man. As touching such locall remedies, which I also daily vsed, were these following,

A digestiue.

℞. Terebinthinæ lotæ in Aqua vitæ ℥. iiii.
Vitellorum ouorum numero ii.
Sir rof. ℥. i.
Mastichis ʒ. i.
Croci q. s.
Misce.

I vsed at euery dressing with this digestiue, to take of Olei rosarum, ℥. i. Mel rosarum ℥. ß. And I dipped the tents and pledgets being warmed, in the said oile and Mel: and after the wound was perfectly digested, then I did mundifie it with this mundificatiue, and such like.

A Mundificatiue.

℞. Terebinthinæ ℥. vj.
Mel rosarum ℥. iiij.
Myrrhæ
Iridis } ana. ℥. iiij.
Aristolochiæ
Farinæ hordei q. s.
Misce.

After the wound was well clensed, then I vsed this incarnatiue with great profit,

℞. Olei

An Incarnatiue.

℞. Olei com. ℥. iiii.
Ceræ nouæ ℥. j.
Terebinthinæ ℥. ß.
Colophoniæ ʒ. ii.
Picis Græciæ ʒ. i.
Thuris, Mastichis ana. ʒ. i.
Croci ℈. i.
Misce.

The rest of the cure I accomplished with other méete and conuenient remedies, which are with vs daily in vse. And so I end this small note, with the true saying of master Doctor *Foster*, who in a learned lecture of Chirurgery, which he did read in the Phisitions colledge in London, said, that the reason why in these daies we do not performe the like famous cures, which were done by the worthy Grecians, and Arabians, and other old and ancient fathers, is for that we do not vse those old and ancient remedies, which daily they did put in practise, to their great credit, worship, and gaine. Moreouer I say, after this patient was cured, fiue yéeres after following, he came to London, partly to sée me, and to giue thanks, in the presence of master *Baily*, and master *Beden*, both Chirurgeons of saint Bartholomewes hospitall in Smithfield, and there in the presence of vs with others, he did shew the places that were wounded, both where the sword went in, and where it went out: since that time I did neuer sée him, neither do I heare whether he be aliue or not, &c.

The cure of a yoong man, which receiued a wound into the right eie, with the point of a dagger. Cap. 22.

There was committed vnto my cure, a yoong man, which receiued a wound into his right eie, with the point of a dagger, so that Cornea, or the horny membrane did fall flat, vpon the christall humor, by reason most part of the white humor Albumineus, issued out of the wound, he had béen in cure with a certaine Surgeon thrée daies, and then I was called vnto the cure of this patient, whom I found greatly pained with inflammation, a sharpe feauer, and want of sléepe, &c. For which causes by good aduise, and diligent circumspection, he was appointed to be let blood, and likewise clisters, and a verytyin diet was administred vnto him, vntill all these accidents were remoued. And for the more speedie mitigating of his paines, there was in like maner applied vpon his necke and shoulders cupping glasses, and on his forehead and temples, this excellent repercussiue medicine,

℞. Emplastrum Diachalcitheos lib. ß.
Olei rosarum ℥.ij.
Succi plantaginis, & } ana. ℥.i.
Solani }
Albuminum ouorum numero ii.
Aceti rosf. q.s.
Misce.

And somtimes I vsed this with like profit,

℞. Olei rosarum ℥.ii.ß.
Omnium Santalorum ℥.ii.
Bol Armenij ℥.ij.ß.
Albuminum ouorum numero ii.
Vini granatorum q.s.
Misce.

And vnto the wound in the eie, I did drop in this remedie warmed,

℞. Mucilag.sem. cydoniorum extractæ in aqua rosarum }
Tragaganthæ } ana. q.s.
Lactis muliebris & }
Albuminis oui }
Misce.

Then ouer that I applied thicke pledgets of fine tow, well wet in this composition following, being warmed a little,

℞. Lactis muliebris }
Vitellorum, & Albuminum oui } ana.q.s.
Succi semperuini, & }
Olei rosarum }
Misce.

With this maner of dressing, I continued six daies, and was constrained three times a day to dresse his eie, & also againe about twelue of the clock at night: for euer as the medicine did grow warme, then the inflammation and paines increased. But after I had got the victory ouer the paine and inflammation, then there did manifestly appeere a certain quantitie of matter, as it were imprisoned, betweene Cornea and Vuea, the which I did remoue, and take away, with this medicament following,

℞. Aqua

℞. Aquæ rosarum ℥.ij.
Vini albi ℥.j.
Sir.rosati solutiui ℥.ß.
Sacchari candi ℥.ii.
Succi fœniculi ℥.ß.
Albuminis oui q.s.
Misce.

After the matter was remoued, then I changed this course, and vsed these remedies following, wherewith the eie was deliuered from all the foresaid accidents,

℞. Tutiæ præparatæ ℥.j.
Aloes succotrinæ ℥.ß.
Camphoræ ʒ.j.
Aquæ rosarum lib.j.ß.
Vini granatorum lib.ß.
Misce.

Powder that which is to be powdered, and mixe all these togither, and seeth them vpon the coles, and reserue them to your vse. Last of all I ended this cure with Mellis virginei, Sacchari candi, Tutiæ præparatæ, Aloes, ana. q. s. After I vsed this alone, and sometimes dissolued in it Aqua rosarum, and at other times in like sort I vsed Collyrium album sine opio, in Lacte muliebri, & Aqua rosarum, ana.q.s. And thus he was healed, of this wound in his eie, by my selfe: oftentimes I haue also cured the like, being ioyned with other Chirurgions in this citie of London: as master *Baker*, one of hir Maiesties Chirurgions, and also master *Banister*, &c. And this may suffice for a breefe note of this cure.

The cure of a certaine Clothier, dwelling neere vnto the north parts of this land, which was dangerously wounded, fower inches in bredth, aboue the left knee, in such sort, that the *Rotula* or round bone of the knee, did hang downe very much: whom I cured as heerafter shall be declared.

Cap. 23.

Not long since, a certaine Clothier, with two of his neighbors and freends, early in the morning, betweene fower and fiue of the clocke, did take their iourney from London, towards the countrey where they did dwell: they had not trauelled fully two miles, but they

they were set vpon by theeues and robbers, who wounded this man very dangerously, as is before declared, and there he was taken, but his neighbors being better horsed, and also cowardly minded, for very feare they ran away, and so caried their owne and his money with them, being about some fower hundred pounds. So presently he returned to London, vnto whom with all expedition I was brought, for that he bled abundantly. Now without further circumstances, at my first comming, I did take out all the blood, which was congealed in the wound: that being done, I did prepare a sharpe and square pointed needle, with a strong euen and smooth silke thred, well waxed, therewith I did take fiue stitches, one good inch distant betweene euery stitch, and I began my first stitch, in the very midst of the wound, for that I did not thinke it good to make the stitches too thick, bicause they do oftentimes stir vp accidents, as paine, and inflammation, &c. Neither was it fit, that the stitches should be set too thin, for then they would not sufficently hold the sides of the wound togither. So when I had orderly performed the stitching of the wound, and leauing a decent place for the wound to purge at, then I applied thereunto, Oleum hyperici cum gummo, and I staied the bleeding with *Galen* his powder: after that I placed aboue the wound, a very good defensatiue to repell and keepe back euill accidents, then with good bolstering and rowling, I finished this first preseruation or dressing. Immediately after, it was demanded of me, what time I would vndertake to cure him: for said they, he is a man of great trade, and doth daily keepe many poore people at worke, and so could by no meanes be long absent from them, &c. And againe, they would further know, if I would warrant to cure him without a maine, or any imperfection vnto his trauelling: To these their vnreasonable demands, I answered breefly, I would make no warrant at all, neither could I set any certaine day or time when he should be made whole: but I told them, I would doe as much as Art could permit me, to the vttermost of my knowledge and skill. And as touching the wound it selfe, I iudged it very dangerous, partly by reason the wound was aboue the knee, and there the musckles being so strangely cut at the very heads of them, and therefore in great danger to be depriued of the action and vse of that member: for that the muscles were the instruments of voluntary mouing. And the danger was the greater, bicause the ligaments which binde the ioints, were likewise separated and cut, whereby insueth greeuous accidents, very hurtful and dangerous, which euils oftentimes foreshew peril of death. All which to them was small pleasure to heare, and therefore they said vnto me, that they would further consider of my sayings, and so I departed: yet expecting

ting my comming againe to the second dressing: but I was preuented, for in the meane time they had conference with diuers Chirurgeons, whereof some were of mine opinion, and some were not. At the last there was brought vnto them, a man which by his owne report had béene a great traueller, and by his diligence in trauelling had attained vnto much learning and skill in Physicke and Chirurgery, neuertheles in all the time of his trauelling, he had neuer learned to speake well. I trust no honest Artist will héere take occasion to mislike my sayings, as certaine Caualiers did not long ago, being in their ruffe and iolitie, most vntruly misconstering my sayings, which I had noted in the margent of the 29. Chapter of this booke, giuing rashly out, that I should there publish all Surgeons that went to the sea were cage birds, but who so pleaseth to peruse the same, shall truly finde that I spake onely against abusers and not otherwise, but belike some falling into dotage and so hauing a guiltie conscience very odly swallowed a hooke which was not laid for them. And I said againe if it be not better looked vnto by authority, many a braue Captaine, Soldier, and Mariner will perish, as Portugall voiage, and other places of seruice of late, can be a true witnes héerein. I speake not as yet against any good and honest Artist, whether he be traueller or not traueller, for I do greatly commend and accept of those trauellers, which by their trauelling doe manifest and shew themselues profitable members in their countrey and common wealth, wherein they do liue and make their abode. Now as touching good and honest trauellers, héere for example sake I will make plaine vnto you: I read that *Hippocrates* himselfe being the prince of Physitions & Chirurgions, and a singular learned man, and brought vp in the schooles of Athens, yet at the age of eightéene yéeres he departed from his study, and so gaue himselfe vnto trauelling through diuers countries and kingdomes, searching what they did know of the nature and properties of hearbs, and of plants: and what experience he had gathered and séene of them, that he did write downe and commit to memory. It is reported, that twelue yéeres he did thus trauell, after which time he returned, and did come vnto the Temple of *Diana* in Ephesus, where he translated all the Tables of medicines that were there before proscribed many yéeres, and put in good order that which was confused, and added many things, which he had found out by experience, as in those Histories doth more largely appéere. Now after his good example and maner of trauelling, or by any other honest and lawfull means, I do not mislike but commend it greatly, crauing now pardon for my long digression, I will héere presently speake of the foresaid magnificent Chirurgeon, vnto whom it was signified, who did first preserue and dresse

Note.

dresse the patient, with the maner and order of my procéedings in dressing, and mine opinion as concerning the danger of his wound. Now in the forefront of his talke, he proudly said whatsoeuer I had spoken he estéemed it little, if the hurt were no worse than he could conceiue and gather by their talke and information, he would warrant to cure him so that the marrow of the bone were not touched with the weapon: all these words were pleasing vnto them, & very thankfully receiued. But to come to the substance of this cure, may it please thée friendly Reader héere to commit to thy memory, that in my absence before I did come vnto the second dressing of this wounded man, he did in scornfull maner as it was said, take off all my medicines from the wound, and likewise did most foolishly cut open all the stitches, condemning me without mercy, saying vnto them all, I was in a wrong boxe as concerning this cure, coloring his absurdities vpon *Marianus*: for the man would many times be breathlesse with alleging of a number of authors to maintaine his impossibilities, who also would haue wounds lie open without stitching. I answere, that all good Authors command to stitch wounds of necessity, otherwise it would cause a great deformitie. But if the good man had meant small wounds in the face, &c. or brused wounds, where the stitches will rot out, or in venemous bitings, or where the wound that is stitched tendeth to impostumation, there to cut open the stitches I hold it profitable, but shortly after he repented, when it was too late, and would haue excused himselfe with noddies had I wist.

Neuer trust a warranter, nor a bosting bragger, a runnagate fugitiue, nor a lying quacsaluer.

So they said, he procéeded about his busines and did powre into the wound his oile or balme, and next applied his plaister, and so did bolster and rowle it vp after his owne fashion and good liking. Which being thus finished, he gaue him in the morning to drink his most rare Quintessence, as he called it. Then after he had thus finished his dressing, I was sent for vnto the patient, and forthwith they did manifest vnto me, that I should not néede to prepare any thing to dresse the patient, for that was don already by one which had warranted to cure him, & that without any maine and in short time, and whose knowledge and skill excéeded ours far: for that by his great learning, & long trauell he had attained to such rare and singular remedies, as no other man in this part of the world had the like for their great and wonderfull vertues. So by means of his foolish perswasion they discharged me: saying, sith neither you, nor other Surgeons more could warrant to cure the patient wounded, we thanke you for your pains, and so we will trouble you no further. Thus I was by him cōdemned of insufficiency, & as it were cosoned also of my patient. I do omit héer to speake of many things which I could obiect against this vaine glorious boaster and praiser of himself, whose

whose swelling words exceeded, as in my former writings I haue more largely spoken of him. And now to enter briefly into this discourse, I say the seuenth day being expired, at sixe of the clocke at night I was sent for again, & very earnestly requested, that I would take the paines to come againe to speake with the patient: the which to do I was very loth, considering what speeches had past before, but when I vnderstood what danger he was in, I went with the messenger: and being come vnto the patient, he said vnto me, with no small griefe of mind: Now I perceiue the difference betweene such hatefull abusers and other good men of your Art: neuerthelesse I pray you hold me excused, for that lewd felow, which now hath hid his head and is gone away, and hath left me in this miserable case, was first commended vnto me by friends of mine, who were also deceiued by him with his vnsauery eloquence, and vaine and fabulous prating: for vnto me saith he, he hath shewed himselfe one of the vilest persons that liueth, and the deepest dissembler: and for that I said I would heere be briefe, I will therefore come vnto the cure, the seuenth day being expired, it was me thought strange to see, that the wound in so short a time should be so sore oppressed with the abundance of euill humors, which at the first he found without paine, or any other euill accident: which after I cured with these mild and familiar remedies following,

A fomentation.

℞. Vini albi lib.ii.
Aquæ vitæ ℥.iii.
Mirrhæ &
Aloes } ana. ℥.i.
Resinæ pini ℥.iiii.
Misce.

All these were boiled ouer a chafingdish of coles, and with warme steuphs I fomented and bathed the wound.

A Digestiue.

℞. Terebinthinæ lotæ in Aqua vitæ ℥.vj.
Vitellorum ouorum numero ij.
Olei Hyperici ℥.j.
Olei lumbricorum ℥.j.ß.
Mellis Rosarum ℥.ij.
Mastichis ℥.ß.
Hordei q.s.
Croci ℈.j.
Misce.

With the said digestiue I vsed also this decocted balme, which did take great effect in this cure,

A Balme.

℞. Olei Terebinthinæ
Olei Rosarum } ana.℥.iiij.ß.
Olei Lumbricorum
Olei Mastichis } ana.℥.iij.
Olei seminis Lini ℥.iij.ß.
Vermium terrestrium ℥.j.
Terebinthinæ claræ ℥.iiij.
Mastichis
Mirrhæ } ana. ℥.ß
Gummi Elemni
Ammoniaci } ana.ʒ.ij.ß.
Sarcocollæ ʒ.j.
Croci ℈.j.
Misce.

Let the Gums be dissolued in viniger, and then adde thereunto Centaurij maioris m. j. After the herbs be bruised, boile all togither in a faire vessell, untill it come to perfection, and ten daies after set it in the sunne. This balme is maruellous good for wounds in the sinewes and ioints, as it full well appéered in this cure. After I had dipped the pledgets, charged with the digestiue in the said balme, then I laid thereon Emplastrum Triafarmacum Mesuæ.

Emplastrum Triafarmacum Mesuæ.

℞. Lithargyrij subtilissime triti
Aceti vini } ana.lib.j.
Olei veterjs lib.ij.
Fiat Emplastrum secundum artem.

And then I annointed the member round about the wound with Olei papaueris & Olei rosarum ana.℥.j. Misce, which being performed and done, I laid ouer this Cataplasma, and so rowled it up according to art,

A cataplasma Clowes.

℞. Folior.rosarum
Maluarum
Violarum } ana.m.ij.
Florum Chamæmeli
& Meliloti } ana.m.i.
Lactucæ m.ß.

Boile all these in a sufficient quantitie of milke, and when they be tender straine them, and adde thereto,
Rad. Altheæ m.ii.
Seminis Lini m.i.
Seminis Fenigræci m.ß.

Make

Make of these a Mucilage with white wine and water, then put in of this Mucilage ℥.vi.and mixe all togither, then lastly adde

Vnguenti nerualis ℥.ii.
Olei Rosarum & } ana.℥.i.ß.
Olei Chamæmeli }
Medullæ panis m. i.
Farinæ hordei q.s.
Vitellorum ouorum numero ii.
Croci ʒ.ß.
Misce, & fiat Cataplasma.

Thus by this maner and order of curing, with conuenient diet, purging and blœding, in a reasonable time his extreme raging paines were greatly appeased, and the inflammation ceased: after that the wound did tend towards digestion, and the patient againe well comforted. Then bicause the wound was very large and wide one part from another, I did make and frame a certaine plaister for dry stitches, which greatly pleasured vs in bringing the borders and sides of the wound togither, which plaister is published in this bœke. Also the accidents being remœued, I left off the vse of the Cataplasma, and in the place thereof applied Emplastrum Diachalcitheos, dissolued in Oleo rosarum & Oleo mirtillorum, &c. And somtimes in like maner I vsed for a defensatiue Albuminum ouorum & Aluminis rochæ, made in very fine powder, and so well laboured togither ana.q.s. and I applied it about the member, and it did profit vs very greatly: since which time I haue sœne it often vsed in the Lowe countries by one *Hadrian*, Graue *Hollocks* Chirurgion, a very skilfull man: and after I did leaue off the vse of digestiues, and in the place thereof I applied Vnguentum apij, sometimes therewith I mixed the yelk of an egge, & also I vsed Vnguentum Resinæ, a very gœd remedie for wounds in the ioints: and with these vnguents I vsed the foresaid decocted balme, ℥.ij. and added thereto of Lipsius ℥.j. So after the wound was hœrewith well mundified, and the accidents remœued, then by the counsell of a learned man both in physicke and chirurgerie, I was aduised to vse Vnguentum Nicotianum, which he said had wrought wonders aboue belœfe, but I found not that excellencie in it, which he promised and I lœked for: neuertheles, I acknowledge it a medicine not to be disallowed: and this is the order of making of it, as the Physitions appointed. ℞. Fol. Nicotianæ lib.j. let the leaues be well stamped, and after strained out as strongly as possible may be, then adde thereto, Ceræ nouæ, Resinæ, Olei comm.ana.℥.iii. let all these boile togither vnto the consumption of the iuice, then adde thereunto Terebinthinæ Venetæ ℥.iii. boile all togither a little, and reserue it to your vse.

M.Keble.

Vnguentum Nicotianum.

But this vnguent since it was first knowen, is greatly bettered, chiefly by *Iosephus Quercetanus*, and other also. After I had left off the vse of Vnguentum Nicotianum, I vsed then Vnguentum Basilicon maiestrale. Now heere is to be noted, that as often as the flesh did growe spungious, then I did rebate the same with Mercurij præcipitati, and often times with Alumen combust. in aceto rosar. and with the saide vnguent I vsed Oleum Apparisij, after this description following,

Oleum Apparisij.

℞. Olei communis veteris lib. iii.
Terebinthinæ abiectiuæ lib. ij.
Vini albi veteris, & electi lib. ß.
Olibani triti lib. ß.
Furmenti purgantis ℥. iiij. vel ℥. vj.
Hyperici lib. ß.
Valerianæ } ana. ℥. iiii.
Cardui benedicti }
Misce.

Infuse the herbes being brused in white wine, six or eight houres, and ad thereunto the wheat and oile, and so melt them at an easie fire, to the consumption of the wine, after straine them, and then put to the Terebinthine, & Olibanum, and so boile them at a soft fire to perfection. I was in the end greatly troubled in the drying or skinning vp of this wound, notwithstanding the vse of Vnguentum desiccatiuum rub. & Vnguentum de minio, or any other whatsoeuer, vntill I had vsed therewith, this remedy following, ℞. Aquæ vitæ ℥. iiii. Aluminis ʒ. iii. Camphoræ ʒ. i. ß. Misce. Thus by the helpe of almightie God, I finished this cure, and he was againe recouered, but the motion perished: for he had the imperfection of a stiffe knee, which constrained him to vse a leather strap, fastened vnto the toe of his shoe, and againe made fast vnto his body, and so he remaineth vnto this day, &c.

The maner and order, of the taking or cutting off a mortified and corrupt leg or arme, which commeth oftentimes, by reason of wounds made with gun shot, &c. Cap. 24.

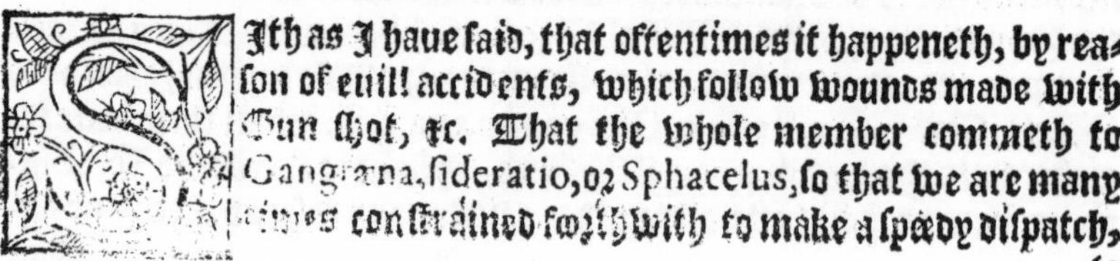

Ith as I haue said, that oftentimes it happeneth, by reason of euill accidents, which follow wounds made with Gun shot, &c. That the whole member commeth to Gangræna, sideratio, or Sphacelus, so that we are many times constrained forthwith to make a speedy dispatch, to

to cut off the member, which shall be don as M. *Gale* & others, very skilfully haue pointed in the whole and sound parts. And if it so fall out, that the leg is to be cut off beneath the knee, then let it be distant from the ioint fower inches, and three inches aboue the knee: and so likewise in the arme, as occasion is offered. These things being obserued, then through the assistance of almightie God, you shall luckily accomplish this worke, by your good industrie and diligence. But you must be very circumspect and carefull of all things, which concerne the methodicall perfection of this worke: that is, you shall haue a great regard to the state of his body, for euacuation and dieting: And after that his body is well prepared and purged, then the same morning you do attempt to cut off the member, be it leg or arme, let him haue some two houres before, some good comfortable caudell, or other broths, according unto the discretion of the Physition, or Chirurgeon, onely to corroborate and strengthen his stomacke, and in any wise omit not, but that he, or shee, haue ministred unto them some good exhortation, concerning patience in aduersitie, to be made by the minister or preacher. And you shall likewise aduertise the friends of the patient, that the worke which you go about is great, and not without danger of death, for that many accidents, and euill symptomes do happen, which in such causes many times do admit no cure: all which being well considered, then ordaine the night before, some good defensatiue, and let it be applied, two or three times about the member,

A defensatiue Clowes.

℞. Emplastrum diachalcitheos lib. i. ß.
Succi semperuiui
Succi plantaginis } ana. ℥. i.
Succi solani
Olei ros. ℥. ii. ß.
Olei mirtini ℥. j.
Ouorum albumium numero ii.
Aceti ros. ℥. i.
Misce.

To the same effect and purpose, I haue in like maner used this defensatiue following, with good successe,

A defensatiue Gale.

℞. Boli Armeniaci ℥. viii.
Farinæ hordei ℥. iiii.
Sanguinis draconis
Terræ sigilatæ } ana. ℥. ii.
Olibani ℥. i. ß.
Aceti ℥. iiii.
Albumin. ouorum q. s. Misce.

All

All which being conſidered, you ſhall haue in a readines, a good ſtrong and ſteady fourme, and ſet the patient at the very end of it: then ſhall there beſtride the fourme behinde him, a man that is able to holde him, or hir faſt, by both the armes: which done, if the leg muſt be taken off beneath the knee, let there be alſo appointed another ſtrong man to beſtride the leg, that is to be cut off, and he muſt hold the member very faſt aboue the place, where the inciſion is to be made, and very ſteadily, without ſhaking, drawing vp the ſkin and muſcles, and he that doth ſo hold, ſhould haue a large ſtrong hand, and a good faſt gripe, whereby he may the better ſtay the bleeding, in the place or ſteede of a ſtraight band, or ligature, which band indeed is alſo very neceſſarie, for, by reaſon of the hard and cloſe binding, it doth ſo benum that part, that the paine of the binding doth greatly obſcure the ſence, and feeling of the inciſion, and the foreſaid band is likewiſe a good direction, for him that doth cut off the member: but yet in ſome bodies, it will not be amiſſe, to admit bleeding, according to diſcretion, ſpecially in ſuch bodies, as are of hot complexions, & do abound in blood, and I haue often ſeene, by the ſkilfulnes of the holder, there hath not been loſt at a time fower ounces of blood: for in weake bodies, it is not good to looſe much blood: for blood is ſaid to be the treaſure of life, and for that cauſe cheefly, a good holder is not to be ſpared. In like maner, there muſt be choſen another ſkilfull man, that hath good experience in holding the leg below, for the member muſt not be held too high, for feare of ſtaying, or choking of the ſawe, neither muſt he beare downe his hand too low, for feare of breaking or fracturing of the bones, in the time it is a ſawing, or cutting off: and he that is the maſter or Surgeon, which doth cut off the member, muſt be ſure he haue a ſharpe ſawe, alſo a very good catlin, and an inciſion knife, and then boldly, with a ſteddy and quicke hand, cut the fleſh round about to the bones, without ſtaying, being ſure the Perioſteum, or pannicle that couereth and compaſſeth the bones, be alſo inciſed and cut, and likewiſe a certaine muſcle or ſinew, that runneth betweene the bones of the leg, which ſhall be done with your inciſion knife: all this being orderly performed, then ſet your ſawe as neere vnto the ſound fleſh, as well you may, & ſo cut aſunder the bones, which done, *Ambroſe Pare*, a man of great knowledge, & experience in Chirurgerie, willeth, preſently after the bones are cut aſunder, that yee then draw the ſides of the wound togither, with fower ſtitches, that are deepe in the fleſh, & made croſſe wiſe, ouer the member, like vnto the letter X for ſaith he, you may eaſily draw the portions of the ſkin, and their diuided muſcles, which before the ſection were drawne vpward, ouer the bones, and couer them cloſe on euery ſide, that they may take the leſſe aire, and the

wound

wound sooner conglutinate, &c. I must confesse I haue cured many, and yet neuer so stitched them: notwithstanding, I wish all men to follow the best way, for the good of their patient. But I say, hauing prepared in a readines this restrictiue, to staie the flux of blood, I procéeded then as followeth,

A restrictiue powder. Clowes.

Rx. Boli Armeniaci ℥.iii.
Sanguinis Draconis, Aloes, ana. ℥.j.
Olibani ℥.i.ß.
Terræ sigillatæ, Mastichis, ana. ℥.i.
Lapidis Hæmatitis ℥.ß.
Calcis ex testis ouorum, Mumiæ, ana. ℥.i.
Gypsi ʒ.vi.
Farinæ volatilis ℥. iiii.
Misce.

Take of this powder as much as will serue your turne, and mixe with the said powder Pilorum leporis, & ouorum albuminum ana. quod satis est, let your Hare haires be the whitest and the softest that is taken from vnder the belly of the Hare, and cut so fine as possible may be, and with the said powder let all be mixed togither, and so brought to a reasonable thicknesse. And note that before yée cut off the member, let there be in like maner made for the purpose, thrée or fower smal bolsters or buttons, fashioned in the top or vpper part like a Doues egge, or as a sugar lofe button, flat in the bottom to the compasse of a French crown, and round vpwards as aforesaid: and these you shall make of very fine towe according to Art, wrought vp in water and vineger, whereupon you shall apply some part of the restrictiue, being mixed as I haue before declared. But yée shall héere further note that one *Gulemew*, a famous Chirurgeon in Fraunce, with other very learned and skilful men, counselleth vs to drawe out the veins and arteries with an instrument called a Rauens bill, and then they tie those vessels with a double strong ligature or thréed, and so safely stay the bléeding, but for that I neuer practised this order by stitching the veins and arteries, I will leaue it as aforesaid, and procéede with mine owne approued practise: and therefore I say when the holder of the member aboue the knée doth partly release the fast holding of his hand, by little and little, whereby you may the better perceiue and sée the mouthes of the veines, that are incised and cut, and vpon those veines, you shall place the round endes of the small buttons, and vpon them presently lay on a round thicke

bed

bed of tow made vp in water and vineger, so that it be fit as néere as you can gesse it, to the compasse of the stumpe or member that is taken off, and thereon spread the restrictiue, and vpon that againe you shall lay another broder bed of towe made vp as you haue heard, so large that it may compasse ouer the member, & that it may be safely tied to kéepe on the rest: wherupon yée shall in like maner spread of the restrictiue reasonable thick, afore yée place it to the rest, and yée shall cut it in fower places, one cut right ouer against another, an inch in length and somwhat more: and yée shall tie or fasten the said large bed to with a ligature, which they call a choke band doubled two or thrée times, being flat and fully an inch brode and a yard long: in the middle of the said ligature or band, you shall spread some of the restrictiue, so that it may take the better hold vnto the large bed of tow, being very fast tied, then you shall place thereon a double large bed of soft linnen cloth, and then with a strong rowler of fower inches brode, and thrée or fower yards long, let it be artificially rowled, and where the blood beginneth to shew, in that place spéedily lay on a good compressor or thicke bolster made of tow wrought vp in water and vineger, the thicknes in the middle to a mans hand, and the thinner towards the edges, in compasse of a Philips dolor, more or lesse, as you suppose the greatnes of the flux to be, and couch them close to, in as many places as the blood doth shew it selfe, and thus with two or thrée rowlers, & as many soft linnen beds, some single, and some double, with a sufficient number of bolsters, some great, and some small you may safely stay the flux of blood: which order and way did neuer faile me, nor any other that haue vsed the same according vnto the order héere prescribed: also sometimes we do vse to draw ouer the great bed of tow being surely tied with the foresaid chokeband, a wet Oxe bladder, and so do pull it close vp ouer the same the which is tied fast also with a ligature or chokeband, and vpon the same a double or single bed of soft linnen cloth, and thus with a few brode bolsters and rowlers very orderly is staied the flux of blood. All which being artificially done, then you shall as easily as possible may be, carie the patient to his bed, hauing a pillow made ready to rest the member on: Thus let him lie with as much quietnes as you can, kéeping a conuenient diet: then the third or fourth day if nothing do let, you shall haue in a readines steuphs of white wine, with decent rowlers, and bolsters and other necessaries as this digestiue following, &c. méete for the second dressing,

A digestiue.

℞. Terebinthinæ in aqua vitæ lotæ ℥.iiii.
Vitellorum ouorum numero ii.
Olei ros. ℥.ß.
Sir ros. ℥.j.

Mastichis

Mastichis ʒ.ii.
Farinæ hordei q.s.
Croci ℈.j.
Misce.

I vse to apply vpon the foresaid digestiue, either a plaister of Flos vnguentorum, or this plaister following,

℞. Resinæ lib.ii.
Ceræ lib. i.
Adipis cerui ℥.iiii.
Gummi elemni lib.ß.
Aquæ vitæ lib.ß.
Succi de peto lib. vi.
Misce.

Emplastrum Hyosciami lutei. Clowes.

Boile al these togither till the iuice be consumed, and then straine it, and make it vp in rowles, so after the wound is well digested, you may then vse this mundificatiue, or any other to the same intent and purpose,

℞. Mellis ℥.x.
Farinæ siliginis, Lupinorum, Hordei — ana.℥.j.
Mirrhæ, Aloes — ana.℥.i.ß.
Succi apii, Absinthii — ana.℥.iii.
Terebinthinæ claræ ℥.ii.
Misce.

A very good mundificatiue.

Also I did vsually incarne the parts with this incarnatiue, or else with that which is of my collection, specified in this booke, &c.

℞. Terebinthinæ, Olei rosati — ana. ℥.vj.
Resinæ pini ℥.iiii.
Gummi elemni ℥.ß.
Ceræ citrinæ ℥.iii.
Misce.

Vnguentum incarnatiuum.

With these incarnatiues, somtimes I mixed Aluminis combusti, being made in very fine powder q. s. And it would then also gently mundifie: which done, I did consolidate and dry vp the parts with Vnguentum desiccatiuum rub. or Deminio, and oftentimes with this desiccatiue following,

℞. Antimonii, Cerusæ — ana.℥.i.

Vnguentum desiccatiuum.

Plumbi vsti
Lithargyri } ana. ℥.ii.
Terebinthinæ
Olei rosati ℥.iiii.
Ceræ albæ ℥.iii.
Misce.

To conclude, yée shall here obserue, that if at any time you haue not of my restrictiue powder in a readines, you may thē vse either *Vigoes* order, to cauterize the place, with a bright cauterizing iron, or else with M. *Gales* powder, which is a most worthy inuention, and better pleaseth the patients, than the hot glowing irons, which are very offensiue vnto the eie. But yet the powder wrought with extreme paine, and made a very great eschar, and by that meanes, the bone hath béen afterwards new cut againe, and so did make a very long worke in some, ere euer they were cured. The powder which I haue here published, is of my inuention, & it neuer causeth paine, but often bringeth with it, a perfect white digestiue matter, which powder, I did kéepe secret to mine own priuate vse, and I did first put it in practise in the Hospitall of saint Bartholomewes, as it is well knowne at this day vnto some of the Surgeons, that then serued with me there, who were present with me at that time, when there was taken off in one morning, seauen legs and armes, where by the assistance and helpe of almightie God we staied all their fluxes of blood, without any paine vnto them, but onely in the compression and close rowling, and tendernesse of the wound excepted. After that time, it was giuen out, and made knowne to diuers Surgeons, that were very desirous to haue it: amongst the rest master *Crowe*, a man of great experience, and knowledge in Chirurgerie, he was very earnest with me for it, which for diuers speciall occasions, I was the more willing to impart it vnto him, but not at his first request, vntill he had séene with his owne eies, the experience and proofe of it. Not many daies after, the Masters of the said hospitall requested me, with the rest of the Surgeons, to go to High-gate, some thrée or fower miles from London, to cut off a maids leg, which they had séene in the visitation of those poore spittle houses: the said leg was so gréeuously corrupted, that we were driuen vpon necessitie, to cut it off aboue the knée, which we did performe by the order before prescribed, and he did sée, we staied the flux, and lost not much aboue fower ounces of blood, and so cured hir within a short time after. Then I gaue him the true maner and order of the making of the said powder. Onely this I am to let you to vnderstand, that since my first collection, I haue added other simples, as Crocus martis, which though it be here left out in this booke vpon purpose,

pose, the powder will be profitable notwithstanding. And afore the publishing abroad of the said restrictiue powder, I did giue and impart the same vnto many good Chirurgeons, which haue béen thankfull for it. But I must néedes say againe, other some haue rewarded me most vnkindly, notwithstanding, I haue knowne they haue vsed it, vnto the profit of their patient, and so credit vnto themselues: neuerthelesse, these could finde in their harts, behinde my backe, to reward euill for good: in stead of thanks, I haue béen back-bitten, and thus I reape for my labor chaffe for corne, ill will and priuate grudge, for curtesies and fréndship offered. Therefore I wish all good Artists, considerately to beware, and take héede vnto whom they impart héereafter their secrets, least they also enter with me into the gap of ingratitude, or the vnsauorie dunghill of despitefull toungs, &c.

The cure of the Gunner of a ship, which was very dangerously wounded, into the lower region of the belly, so that a great part of the Zirbus, or Omentum, did come out of the wound, with some of the intestines and guts likewise. Cap. 25.

A Gunner of a ship cured of a wound in his belly.

I Haue thought it good fréndly Reader, héere particularly in this Chapter, to set downe the cure of a Gunner of a ship, which was wounded in the belly, as aforesaid, who came vnto me, hauing his guts ready to come forth of the wound, with the zirbus hanging out: Then I caused him to lie downe on a bed vpon his backe, and after diligent search made, I found the guts safe, & not touched of the weapon, then with a strong double thréd, I did tie fast the zirbus as close vnto the woũd as possible wel I might, & within a finger bredth or there abouts I did cut off that part of the zirb that hanged out of the wound, and so I cauterized it with a hot iron almost to the knot: all this being done, I put againe into the body that part of the zirb which I had fast tied, and I left the péece of the thréd hanging out of the wound: which within fower or fiue daies after, nature cast forth the thréd as I say, being fast tied, then presently I did take a néedle with a double strong silke thréd waxed, wherewith I did thrust through both Mirach and Ziphach on the right side of the wound, but on the left side of the wound, I did put the néedle but through Mirach onely, and so tied these thrée fast togither with a very strong knot, and presently I did cut off the thréd, then one

 the

the same side where I did stitch but Mirach onely, which héere I call the the left side, I did there begin againe to thrust the néedle through both Mirach and Ziphach, and also on the right side where I did first begin to force the néedle through Mirach and Ziphach, there I did thrust that but through Mirach onely, and so as before, I made another strong knot, and then I cut off againe the thréed, and after the same maner I made the third stitch, &c. all which is according to *Weckers* and other learned mens opinions & practises, who also say, that the stitches of the one side must be higher than on the other side. After I had thus finished all the said stitches that were there requisit and néedfull to be made, then I did preserue the said wound with the oile of Hyperici, conuaying it in with a fine péece of lawne dipped in the foresaid oile, and so put it into the dependant part of the wound: then to restaine the blœding I placed vpon the wound *Galens* powder, which I mixed with the whites of egs and hare haires, and about the wound I vsed that defensiue, which I haue published in the 23. chapter of this bœke being of my discription: then with gœd bolstring and rowling he rested till the second day. Yée shall moreouer vnderstand, that immediatly after he did complaine of the grudging of an ague, and being therewith somewhat distempered, presently there was a veine opened, and a gentle mollifieng clister also administred, whereupon he amended very shortly after: and thus his feuer was preuented. The third day we opened the wound, and found it without paine, or any other euill accident: then the first thing was done, I fomented and bathed the wound with this wound drink, which is of my collection,

A wound drinke. Clowes.

℞. Vini albi lib. viii.
Aquæ com. lib. x.
Sacchari albi lib. ii.
Consolidæ vtriusque
Filicis aquaticæ
Calendulæ
Ophioglossi
Chelidonij
Polipodii quercini
Numulariæ
Lilij conuallium
Sanimundi
Diapensiæ
Veronicæ
Verbenæ
Pimpinellæ } ana. m. i.

Let

Let these herbs first lie and digest in the wine and water for the space of fower daies, and after boiled in Balneo mariæ, but let the vessell wherein the ingredients are be wel luted & stopped with very good past, that none of the vapors & substance passe forth, and so reserue it to your vse. Sometimes in stéed of sugar I do put in of clarified hony the like quantity, and it doth worke wonderfull well: which done I did put into the wound being warmed, the oile of Hypericon, with a péece of fine lawne: herewithall I administred Vnguentum de peto, or Nicotian, being dipped in the said oile warme, & laid vpon the same the gum plaister with warme double steuphs dipped in the said wound drinke, and wrong out againe, and then rowled it vp according to Art. Then presently in the morning I gaue him to drinke fower ounces of the saide wound drink, and about thrée or fower of the clocke in the after noone, I gaue him fower ounces more, and about seuen or eight of the clocke at night, I gaue him other fower ounces, and thus I continued this course till he was cured. Likewise for a time his ordinary drinke at meals was ptisanes & barly water, and he was moreouer adioined to a thin & cooling diet: and so by this maner and order of dressing both morning and euening, within the space of one and twenty daies he was perfectly healed.

Also in *Anno* 1580. there was remaining about this city of London, a seruing man called *William Mouch*, who receiued a wound with a sword into his belly, so that the zirb issued out of the wound more broder in compasse than a great trencher, which after was also cured as beforesaid by me and Master *William Crowe* Chirurgion of London.

William Mouch cured of a wound in his belly.

Moreouer, in *Anno* 1586. there was a wench about the age of ten or twelue yéeres, dwelling with one master *Bracy* a Marchant of London, which wench was also wounded in the belly with a knife which she caried in hir hand, and without regard running ouer hastily she fell vpon the same knife, so that the zirb did come out of the wound more than the compasse of a mans hand, she then being in the countrey about seauen miles from London: vnto whom I was intreated to go, so I went, and presently at my comming, I did cut off that part of the zirb that hanged out of the wound, and then I tied it fast, as before I haue said. But you shall truly héere vnderstand, I did not vse any cautrize vnto this wench, neither yet vnto the seruingman aboue named, the reason was, for that the patients & their friends also, could not abide to heare the cauterizing irons named, although I confesse if the pains were excepted) there is no way comparable: notwithstanding I found this order aforesaid most certaine and sure. Which yong maiden was after brought to London, whom I likewise did cure in a very short time within the city of London, and she liueth at this day.

A wench cured of a wound in hir belly.

Now

Now to finish and ende these obseruations before declared, I thinke it needfull, that I speake also briefly of the maner and order of diet and purging, which the patient wounded for the most part onght to follow, the which *Tagaltius* and *Guido* with other learned men haue published, and is requisite to be obserued, especially where the learned Physitions are not to be had at the seas, in great and long voiages. Cap. 26.

Order of dieting.

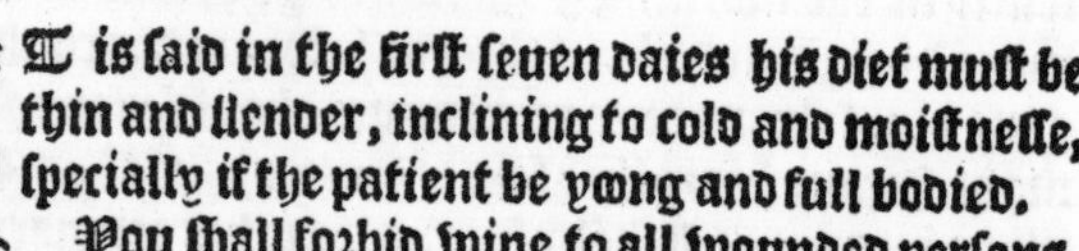

IT is said in the first seuen daies his diet must be thin and slender, inclining to cold and moistnesse, specially if the patient be yong and full bodied.

You shall forbid wine to all wounded persons, chéefly if they haue a feauer, and incline to an inflammation.

Let them abstaine from all flesh that is hard and tough, and from great fishes that engender euill iuice, also from new and vnleauened bread, euill made and baked.

Also it is good to refraine from all chéese, and chéefly that which is old and salt, from fruits almost of all sorts, from garlike, onions: all sharpe and salt things, and let him not taste of any kinde of hot spices.

He may vse partriges, pullets, and birds that haunt the woods: let them haue ptisanes of barley and almond milke, and vse potage made with flesh of veale, simple or prepared with egs.

Let him haue lettice, purslane, borage, buglosse, spinage, and such like herbs in broths.

His drinke shall be water boiled, wherein is soked houshold bread, such as hath some part of bran in it, commonly called browne bread, or in the stead of the said water, let him drinke a ptisan of barly: or if he be weake or old, let him drinke tart and stipticke wine, allaied with plentie of water and sugar.

His supper must be short, yet nourishing.

It is good to vse light and gentle rubbing or chafing of the parts, somwhat far off from the wounded part.

Let him be quiet: for quietnes is his chiefe medicine, and stirring and walking contrarie, especially if he be wounded in the lower parts of the bodie.

It

It is necessarie altogither to abstaine from the vse of carnall copulation. And also to shun ire, contention, anger, wrath, and all vehement motions of the minde.

After the seuen daies, when the patient séemeth to be sure and safe from inflammation, and all other euil accidents, then let him vse a more plentifull diet, and by little and little, let him returne to his former custome, and then vse some wine, but weake and gentle: and let him eate such flesh as doth engender good blood, and is a maintainer of naturall heat and moisture, and the strength of the bodie: such as is the flesh of hens, capons, and mutton, especially the mutton of weathers: and this diet is necessarie and commodious to wounded men, bicause it maintaineth the naturall habite of the body, and doth not moue or stir vp feauers, inflammations, or fluxes: And to this kinde of diet, saith *Tagaltius*, do all the best Physitions and Chirurgions agrée, as *Galen*, *Hali*, *Rhasis*, *Auicen*, *Brunus*, *Lanfrancus*, and *Guilielmus de Saliceyto*, yet *Theodoricus* and *Henricus* are of a contrarie opinion: for they would haue wine and hot diet, to be giuen and vsed immediately vpon the wound receiued: for (say they) the weaknes of the faculties of the wounded person, is by and by to be strengthened and confirmed, and that by the drinking of wine: whose sentence and iudgement is repugnant to reason, as *Galen* j.lib.& Aphoris.iiii.saith: it chanceth but seldome in sicknesses, that we should studie to restore the strength of the body more than it may receiue: for in so doing we shall increase and maintaine the sicknes. So that it appéareth by *Galens* words, that we must not alwaies hasten to increase the strength, but it is sufficient somtimes to conserue and maintaine the same: so that from the first time that the wound is receiued to the seuenth day, in the which time inflammations vse to come, let the vse of drinking wine be altogither forbidden, vnles through flux of blood the strength be greatly inféebled. *Celsus* saith, ye may refresh the patient a little with wine, but otherwise it is an enimie to wounds. After the seuenth day, if nothing do let, vse wine allaied with water: for if the wound remaine without accidents till then, it is commonly afterward in safetie. Therefore nothing (I say) héerein can be more necessary for a yoong practiser in Surgerie, than to indeuour himselfe to knowe before what euill will follow, and to learne how to preuent it. And thus much I haue collected, concerning dieting of your patients: being (as I said) at the sea in great and long voiages, or in the wars by land, where the learned physition is not alwaies at hand to be had, for helpe and counsell héerein, for which causes I haue héere set downe in like sort, a very short and briefe note, for the maner and order of purging of your patients. Ye shall further vnderstand, if the patient wounded be bound

in

in his belly, and not laxatiue: for remedie thereof you may vse a clister, or a suppositorie, or else giue the patient Cassia, or Manna, or some such gentle purging medicine: but if he be of an euill habit or complexion, and so replenished with euill iuice, or if the wound be greeuous and great, yea though his bodie were pure and cleane, yet those gentle purgings will not then suffice, but we must vse stronger medicines: so that there are two principall obseruations in purging of your patients, in such wounds the greatnes of the greefe, and the abundance of the euill iuice. But if the wound consist in the vpper part of the bodie, then to purge downward is the counsell of the learned, and if the wound be in the lower parts of the bodie, to stay the flux of humors from flowing thither, it is meete and conuenient to withdraw the same by purging or vomiting, which is to be done with great discretion. Thus much as it were in a word, I haue thought it not amisse to note and obserue, out of these learned authors before spoken of, which in my practise in curing I haue followed, and it is at this day ratified and confirmed by diuers learned Physitions and Chirurgions, &c.

Order of purging.

Next followeth a note of certaine necessarie medicines and instruments, good for yoong practisers of Chirurgerie to be furnished with, which follow the wars either by sea or land.

Cap. 27.

It is most truly said, there is no coine so currant, but hath in it some counterfaits, which make it suspitious: so is there no profession so good, but hath also some counterfaits, which breede in it disgrace, and none so much (I suppose) as there are some in these daies, that take vpon them the honest titles & names of trauelling Surgeons, nay these are idle and ignorant menslaiers, or wandring runnagate surgeons, that I speake of, which very boldly with most glorious facings, challenge vnto themselues to be the onely masters of Chirurgery in the world, bicause they haue a little trauelled: neuerthelesse, a number of these od, arrogant, & friuolous fellowes, are knowne to be men altogither ignorant in the art, both in reason, iudgement, and experience, howbeit, some one of them will vse more comparisons, prating and babling words, than fower wise men would willingly answer: and you shall also farther know them by this note: They are most commonly vnfurnished of all good medicines, either medicinal, or instrumentall, vnlesse it be some such palterie stuffe, which a man would

Many good ships are as it were, become cages for such vnclean birds the more is the pitie.

would scarce lay to a gauld horse back, with other furniture answerable to the same. And so they are no more able to performe any good cure they take in hand, than they be able with one puffe of their winde to turne about a milstone, for their cures at their comming home, are plaine demonstrations of their beastly ignorance, and thus they bring themselues into ignominie and shame, and the worthy artist into very great discredite. Therefore fréendly Reader, let this be a warning vnto thée, to take héede of these vncleane birds, who do daily abuse many worthy persons, Captains, Gentlemen, Masters of ships, and Marchants of good account, by reason of the shamelesse braggings, and boastings of their great diuine magnificent skils in Physicke and Surgery, wherewith they say they are adorned, and excéede all others, vnder colour hereof, by their fraude and subtill meanes, they haue béen & daily are entertained to be principall surgeons for great ships of war, and charge of numbers of men: and hauing receiued aforehand, towards the preparation and furnishing of their surgerie chests, of some twenty pounds, and of some fortie and fiftie pounds: but in conclusion, they falsified their promises, for shortly after they had receiued their money, they lay a loofe of, lurking for opportunitie, and so in the end ran away, and could not be found nor heard of, vntill the captaines that hired them, had set saile and gone forewards one their great & long voyages, without any surgeon at all. But good Reader, what hath insued hereof: truly many a braue soldier and mariner hath perished, and sometimes the Generall and Captaines themselues, and so by this meanes, partly the whole voyage hath béen ouerthrowne, by reason they had no helpe or succour, either of Physicke or Surgerie to reléeue or comfort any of them. But what remedie or redresse I know not, they are no changlings, for still they perseuere in their wickednes, without check or controlment. The like broode of abusers and abuses, I read of in some sort in a certain history, which lately came vnto my hand, and it is published in the French toung, by a most famous Surgeon in France, one *Gulemew*, Surgeon to the French King, and it is written by him in the apologie to his last booke in Surgery, fol. 134. The common discourse saith " he, of Chirurgery, or Surgery, at this day is more vaine fabulous, " and imaginatiue, than the birth of the gods, the history of the giants, and " the studie of the philosophers stone, with a thousand other phantasticall " deuises: there is reported saith he, that there is but one good Surgeon " in all France, which euery one thinketh he hath: from whence is " commonly said, I haue the best Surgeon of the world, so that some of " them will vaunt of a thousand absurdities and impossibilities, some " one will say, by his spéedie industrie and exquisite knowledge, that he "

„ will cure a man that is wounded through the head, in the turning of a „ hand or a moment, though the braines come out: another will say, that „ he will heale and cure a man of his sight, though his eie be stricken out „ of his head, and fall to the earth, without any blemish to the sight, or „ without any danger of death: another saith, that he will cure a man, „ that is striken through the hart with a caliuer shot, or through any part „ of the body, &c. Many other absurdities he wisely noteth of such notable liers and shamelesse braggers, who, (as I haue spoken of before,) do abuse many notable men, with their vaine promises and impossibilities. But what remedy I know not, for most commonly I sée, the basest sort of Surgeons are accounted for the best, and the best, for the basest. To conclude, I haue here for the benefit of all yong practisers in Chirurgerie, collected out of *Iosephus Quercitanus*, and also out of *Vigo*, with others, certaine speciall medicines and necessary instruments: whereunto, I haue also added somewhat of mine owne collection, very néedefull and necessary for all those Chirurgions to be furnished with, which follow the wars either by sea or land: vnto whom I wish most happie and good successe, as vnto my selfe, as knoweth God, the true witnesse and iudge of all men.

Iosephus Quercetanus.

Suppuratiues or maturatiues are said to be,

Vnguentum basilicon vtriusque.
Vnguentum Macedonicum.
Tetrapharmacum.
Vnguentum resumptiuum.

The emplaister of Mucilages, may be dissolued with oile oliue, if néede require.

Mundifying and clensing medicines,

Vnguentum diaphompholygos Nicolai.
Vnguentum viridis Andromachi.
Emplastrum diminio dissolued in oile of roses.
Vnguentum apostolicum Auicennæ.
Vnguentum Ægyptiacum Auicennæ.

Incarnatiues or regeneratiues,

Vnguentum Aureum.
Vnguentum ceraseos Mesuæ vtriusque.
Emplastrum de Gratia Dei, & de Ianua.

Desiccatiues or drying medicines,

Vnguentum Deminio.

Vnguentum

Vnguentum desiccatiuum rub.
Emplastrum de cerusa.

Unguents for burnings with gun powder,
Vnguentum Fuscum Nicolai.
Vnguentum calce viua.
Vnguentum Maistrale of the Phisitions of Florence, descri-bed by *Weckerus*.

Medicines to repell and keepe backe,
Vnguentum de bolo communi.
Vnguentum rosarum Mesuæ.

Of syrupes these be conuenient,
Acetosus simplex. Vigo.
A syrup of the iuice of Endiue, or
De duabus radicibus, without vineger.
Mel rosarum, in small quantitie.

Waters these shall suffise,
Water of Endiue.
Hops.
Borage.
Wormwood.
Fumitory, of euery one a sufficient quantitie.

Of Electuaries, they shall haue with them,
Diaphenicon.
Elec. de succo rosarum after Mesua.
Diacatholicon.
Cassia.

Pils they must haue.
Pillulæ hieræ cum agarico.
Pillulæ fumariæ, the greater and the lesse.

Against the disease Ophthalmia, they must haue,
Aqua rosarum, and a siefe without Opium.

Oyles are these,
Olea. Rosaceum.

Myrtillorum.
Chamæmelinum.
Ompharinum.

And it is conuenient, that they haue with them also,

Clowes.

Farinæ.

Farinæ.	Fabarum Orobi Lini Fœnugræci Hordei Lupinorum Tritici	ana. q. s.

Emplaisters.

Emp. de speciebus.
Emp. diachalcitheos.
Emp. cum gummo.
Emp. sticticum Paracelsi.
Emp. hyoscyami lutei Clowei.
Emp. Cumini.
Emp. floris vnguentorum.
Em. Deminio.

Vnguents.

Vnguentum dialthææ.
Vnguentum album Rhasis.
Vnguentum depeto, or nicotian.

Arceus liniment for wounds in the head, and his plaister for the same,

Vnguentum prospasma.
Balsamum artificiale.
Oleum Hyperici cum gummo.
Oleum Catulorum.
Oleum Lumbricorum.
Oleum Ouorum.
Oleum Scorpionum.
Oleum Amygdalarum dul.
Butyrum recens.

A lotion for sore mouthes méet for such as haue the scorby, which oftentimes falleth out at the sea, and likewise by land, for the true cure of it I refer

refer you to *Wyerus*, which booke is translated of late into English. But in steed thereof read the 12. chapter of this booke, where you shall be partly satisfied.

Mithridatum, or fine Treacle.
Sperma ceti.
Also french barly.
Licoris.
Aniseeds likewise to be remembred.
Potus Antiochiæ, or some other good wound potion, that will last a long time for wounds in the body.

For Cataplasmes or Poultises, yee shall cary with you,

Flores.
Ros.
Chamæmel.
Meliloti in pul.
Rad. altheæ in pul.

To rebate and take away spungious flesh,

Mercurii præcipitati.
Mercurii sublimat.
Alumen rochæ.
Vitriolum.

Also take with you,

Eggs.
Towe.
Vineger.
Splints for fractured or broken bones.
Tape to binde on the splints.
Cupping or boxing glasses.
A chafingdish.
A morter and a pestle.

Restrictiue powders to restraine great fluxes of blood,

Galens powder.
Gales powder.
Clowes powder.

Small and long ware candles to search the hollownes or depth of a wound.
Also long probes made of siluer, tin, lead, or wood.

Needles

Néedles two or thrée, some eight inches, some ten or twelue inches in length, hauing a decent eie in it guttered like a spanish néedle, and the point or end blunt or round, that it offend not in the going in of it, made fit to draw a Flammula or a péece of fine lawne or linnen cloth through the body or member that is wounded.

Moreouer you must carie with you,

A sharpe sawe.

A faire large catlin to cut the flesh vnto the bones.

Likewise a fine incision knife.

Also small buttons, or cauterising irons méete to stay the flux of an artery or vaine, if great necessity require it.

A trepan.

A head sawe.

An eleuatory.

A dilatorium to open a wound that a dart head, arrow head, or bullet, may the better be taken out.

With a rostrum Coruinum, or Rauens bill.

Or with a rostrum Anatinum, or Ducks bill.

Or with a rostrum Gruinum, fashioned like a Storks bill or Cranes bill.

There be in vse of these two sorts, the one bowing, and the other straight.

A speculum Oris, for the mouth.

A syring.

As for stitching quils and other instruments, that a Surgion ought alwaies to cary about him, I leaue vnspoken of.

There are also many other instruments I know which are in vse, but these may suffice which I haue here descibed in the end of this booke, for yong students and practizers in the Art, and vnto men of great experience and iudgement, it is néedlesse for me to nominate the rest.

Now followeth other approoued remedies for wounds in generall, but specially for wounds made with Gun shot. Cap. 28.

OLeum catulorum practised in the Lowe Countries for wounds made with Gun shot, &c. by one master *Iohn Burioice* a french Surgion, who serued vnder the Lord *Willoughby*, which oile as it may appéere, was first published by master *Ambrose Pare*, whereunto some haue added of late these herbes following, which thing no doubt procéeded

procéeded from men of good iudgement and experience. But other gréene heads for want of knowledge of the excellency of the said oile, do little estéeme of it, by reason of their brutish iudgement: but they are to be regarded, as réeds shaking in the winde. This oile was sent vnto me for a singular secret, out of the Lowe Countries by one M. *Iames* a Surgion dwelling in Utrick, & I haue also proued it a most worthy remedy, &c.

R. Olei vitel. lib.iiij.
Catulos duos
Vermium terrestrium lib.j.

Boile these ouer a gentle fire of coles till the flesh be separated from the bones, then straine them, & ad thereto Terebinthinæ Venetiæ ℥.iiii. Aquę vitæ ℥.i. Some as héereafter shall be declared, haue added vnto this oile these herbes following, which they say profit greatly: the leaues of Nicotian iiij. handfuls, the leaues of Ribwort, the leaues and rootes of Comfery, of each a handfull and a halfe, shred all these, and after they be stamped, then put them into the oile, and so let it rest sixe daies, and then boile it with the rest of the ingredients, and boile all till the iuice be consumed. But to speake truly, I haue vsed it without addition, as Master *A. Pare* hath published, which for the excellency thereof, I cannot but commend so much, as it worthily deserueth: for being sent for by letters from the right honorable, and also by hir Maiesties commandement, to go into the Lowe Countries to attend vpon the Earle of Leicester, Lord Liestenant and Captaine generall of hir Maiesties forces in the Lowe Countries: shortly after my comming thither, I was commanded by his Honor, to haue a great regard vnto the preseruing and curing of the hurt and wounded soldiers: and there was also appointed with me in that seruice, Master *Godorus* Sergeant Surgeon vnto hir Maiestie, whose industries and practise did greatly differ from the bitter experiments of a sort of straglers, that did thrust themselues into Captaines bands, for principall masters in Surgerie. But héere to the praise of almightie God, there was not one of our hurt patients, that did at any time complaine of any paine or gréefe, by reason of the application of our remedies, but they did take their naturall rest, being no otherwise shot, but through the thigh, leg or arme, or other fleshie parts of the body, so that no ioints were wounded, or bones greatly fractured, and broken withall: to conclude (I say) being but wounded in the fleshie parts of the body, then our order was first to draw a Flammula through the wounded member, being made of fine lawne, or some other fine linnen cloth, and vpon the same we applied this digestiue, and so stéeped it in the said oile of Whelpes,

Oleum catulorum. A. Pare.

Notæ.

R. Tere-

A digestiue for Gun shot. Clowes.

℞. Terebinthinæ lotæ in Aqua vitæ ℥.iiij.
Vitellorum ouorum numero ij.
Vnguenti Populei simp. ℥.ij.
Olei rosarum ℥.ß.
Mercurij præcipitati ʒ.ii.
Croci ℈.j.
Misce.

As I haue said, after we had conuaied into the wound the said Oleum catulorum being warmed, then into the lower orifices of the saide wound, we did put in a short tent also armed with the digestiue, and so likewise dipped into the oile, and then vpon the same we laid either Emplastrum Hyosciami lutei, or some other such like, and then round about the wounded member, the defensiue made of Emplastrum Diachalcitheos, with the iuices, (as is before set downe in this booke) and then with conuenient rowlings and bolsterings, we accomplished this first preseruation: and when the wound came to perfect digestion, then we did mundifie and clense the parts somtimes with this mundificatiue, or the like, as occasion was offered vnto vs,

A very good mundificatiue. Franciscus Raffius.

℞. Butyri recentis lib.ij.
Ceræ Citrinæ
Resinæ
Resinæ Pini
Picis Græcæ } lib.ß.
Viridis æris ℥.ß.
Misce.

The wound being well mundified and clensed, then we did leaue the vse of the Flammula, and vsed short and easie tents: and after did incarnate, and heale it vp oftentimes with this vnguent following, or such other like, as we thought most méete and conuenient,

Vnguentum consolidatiuum.

℞. Gummi Elemni
Opopanacis } ana.℥.vj.
Bdellij ℥.ß.
Resinæ Pini ℥.j.
Terebinthinæ ℥.iiij.
Thuris
Mastichis } ana.ʒ.ij.
Ceræ citrinæ
Olei Rosarum } ana.℥.x.
Misce.

Moreouer, as occasion serued, if the wound did passe into the bodie, then many times I did iniect into the wound Oleum Hyperici cum gummo,

gummo, and did giue them alſo to drinke, ſome wound drink, ſuch as héerafter ſhall be publiſhed.

A digeſtiue for Gun ſhot.

℞. Mercurij præcipitati biſcalcinati ℥.j.
Butyri recentis ℥.iiij.
Vnguenti Baſilici ℥.iij.
Olei Liliacei & Lini } ana.℥.j.
Camphoræ ʒ.ij.diſſoluti in Aqua vitæ q.s.
Miſce, & fiat vnguentum.

A digeſtiue for Gun ſhot.

℞. Vnguentum Baſilicon ℥.ij.
Butyri recentis ℥.j.
Mercurij præcipitati ʒ.ij.ß.
Miſce,& fiat vnguentum.

An oile for wounds made with gunſhot. Landrada.

℞. Olei Lini lib.ij.
Terebinthinæ lib.ij.
Viridis æris pul.ʒ.ij.
Miſce.

A very good wound drinke practiſed by *Madam Donuill*, which was firſt commended vnto me by Noblemen, Captaines, and ſoldiers, who ſerued in the wars in France. This Lady for hir charitable déeds in the curing of a many wounded ſoldiers, may well be compared vnto *Artemiſia* Quéene of Halicarnaſſus, and wife vnto *Mauſolus* King of Caria: ſhe was the firſt that found out that herbe, which we call in Engliſh Mugwort, the Latine name is after hir owne name Artemiſia.

A wound drinke.

℞. Baccarum lauri
Ariſtolochiæ rotundæ } ana.ʒ.j.
Prunellæ.

Madam Donuill.

Beate all theſe to fine powder, and take of Prunellæ that groweth in the ſhade, then take the fleſh of freſh water Creuiſes dried into powder, and of ſwéete Drace, of ech halfe a dram: tie all theſe togither in a dry linnen cloth, and ſéeth them with a handfull of Vinca peruinca in thrée quarts of white wine till a quart be conſumed. Epithemate the wound, then cloſe the lips of the wound, and couer it with a leafe of red Colewort dipped in the ſaid wine, & lay vpon them large linnen clothes dipped alſo in the ſame wine: likewiſe if the wound be déepe, ſyring in the decoction euery morning & euening, and procéede in the reſt as before: furthermore let him drinke ℥.i.or ii. euery morning, faſting vpon it thrée or fower howers from all meate: if the potion ſéeme too bitter, to the quantity of powders and herbes ad double the quantity of wine,&c.

Or this,

A wound drinke. D.F.

℞. Fol.& rad. rubiæ tincto
Rad.Aristoloch.long.
& rotundæ
Fol.& rad.plantag.
Fol.& rad.consolidæ maioris
& minoris
Fol.& rad.gariophill.
Fol.& rad.centaurii maioris } ana. m.ii.
Rad.altheæ
Summitatum rub.
Summitatum lapathi acuti
Tanaceti
Millefololii
Pimpinellæ
Artemisiæ
Summitatum canubis
Caulis rub.
Fragariæ } ana.m.i.
Thuris albi ℥.ij.
Sarcocollæ ℥.j.
Vini albi Bocalia xv.

Put all these togither in an earthen vessel well nealed or glassed, that halfe the vessell may remaine empty, and let it be close couered, that no aire do euaporate & so boile them for thrée howers with indifferent fire, and let them be strained: vnto the which let there be added Mellis six pound, then let them be boiled again vnto the consumption of the fourth part: the quantity héere is to be giuen in the morning fower ounces, and as much at night: & the wound is to be bathed in the same, laying thereon a Colewort leafe. This said wound drinke is reported to be singular good for the curing of Fistulas: other hidden vertues it hath for curing of wounds, &c. which drinke I obtained of *Doctor Foster*, reader of the Surgery lecture in the Physitians Colledge in London, a man who for his great paines and learned iudgement in the Art, meriteth of vs, which professe Chirurgery, great praises and thanks for his kindnes daily offered.

Or this,

A good wound drink.

℞. Dentis Leonis.
Bugulæ.
Saniculæ.
Cariophillatæ.

Absinthii.

Absinthii.
Abrotani.
Quinque neruiæ.
Betonicæ.
Summitatum rubi.
Consolidæ med.
Consolidæ minoris.
Rad.symphyti.
Rad.liqueritiæ.
Of euery one of these herbes a good handfull.
Prunorum maturorum num.xl.
Vini albi lib.iiii.
Mellis lib.j.vel lib.ß.

Let these be infused twelue howers being well brused, and after boile them til the one part be consumed, &c. who was the author of this wound drinke I could neuer learne: It was giuen vnto me for a speciall thing: and if it were ten times better, I would héere publish it to the good of others: although I know a number are not of my minde and opinion héerein.

Among many other things in the Art of Surgery, this Balme following is greatly to be praised for the curing of gréene wounds, &c.

This Balme is approoued precious in gréene wounds, and healeth them very spéedily and effectually, it healeth scabs & wheales in the face and hands, and causeth them to be very faire: it is excellent in wounds of the sinewes and ioints, it staieth the mucilage and gléeting water: but if you will distil it according to Art, you shall first haue an excellent water: secondly a most pure oile: thirdly the Balme which is most excellent in wounds and vlcers of the fundament. The oile is precious against all aches and gouts, the water also preserueth from venome and pestilence, &c. This Balme was first giuen vnto me, as it is héere described word for word, by one master *Bactor* a practiser of Physick and Chirurgery, which at that time serued the Lord of Aburgauenny, vnto whom I also did retaine, where I sawe the first experience and proofe of this before. But to say truly, who was the first Author or inuentor of it, I do not certainly know: but as I haue hard some say, it is supposed to haue béene deuised by one master *Iohn Hall* Chirurgeon of Maidstone, a most famous man. The composition as followeth, A very good Balme.

℞. Agrimoniæ
Alchimellæ } ana.m.j.
Androsæmi

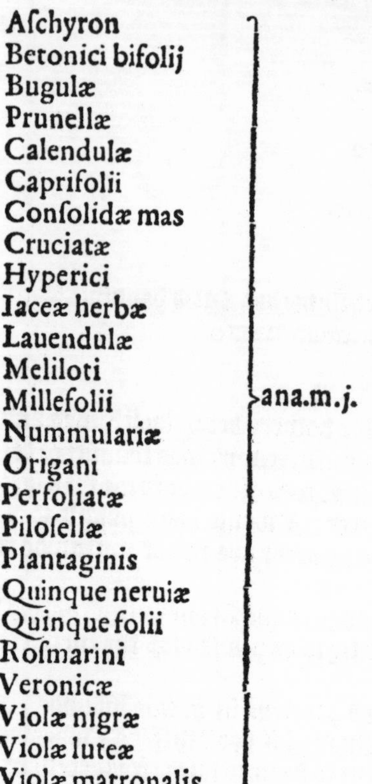
Aſchyron
Betonici bifolij
Bugulæ
Prunellæ
Calendulæ
Caprifolii
Conſolidæ mas
Cruciatæ
Hyperici
Iaceæ herbæ
Lauendulæ
Meliloti
Millefolii
Nummulariæ
Origani
Perfoliatæ
Piloſellæ
Plantaginis
Quinque neruiæ
Quinque folii
Roſmarini
Veronicæ
Violæ nigræ
Violæ luteæ
Violæ matronalis

} ana.m.j.

Let theſe herbes be gathered each one in his time and kinde, and let them be ſtamped, and then put into ſwæte oile oliue, ſo that you may get theſe herbes from time to time, you may in the end haue a gallon of oile to the quantitie of herbes: then let them ſtand togither the ſpace of one moneth in a pot well nealed, and cloſe couered, burie it in hoꝛſe dung, and in the meane ſeaſon get theſe gums following,

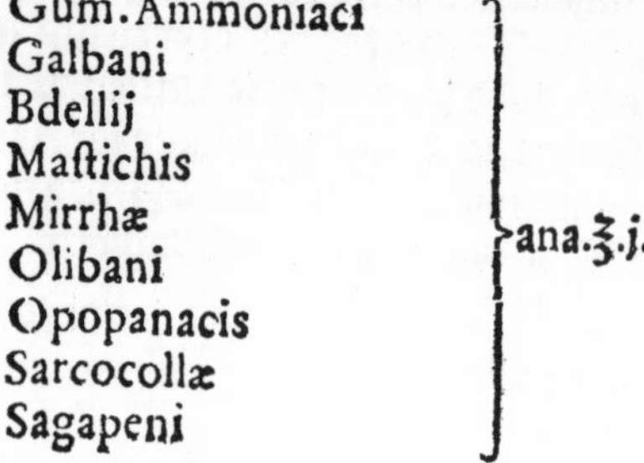
Gum. Ammoniaci
Galbani
Bdellij
Maſtichis
Mirrhæ
Olibani
Opopanacis
Sarcocollæ
Sagapeni

} ana.℥.j.

Storacis

Storacis Calamitæ } ana. ℥.j.
Thuris

Gariophyllorum } ana ℥.j.ß.
Maceris
Nucis muscatæ
Cinnamomi

Powder them that are to be powdered, and dissolue the Gums in good white wine, then set the herbes to the fire in a faire brazen vessell to boile with the oile, putting thereto fower pound of good wine muscadell, of Vermium terrestrium well washed in white wine, and mundified from the earth, thrée pound: let them boile thus togither, stirring them diligently with a slice at a soft fire, till the wine and the iuices be wasted, and that the oile haue a faire gréene colour of the herbes, then let them be strongly strained, and put thereto your gums and other things, togither with fower pounds of odoriferous wine, that is, muscadell or malmsey: then adde thereto Terebinthinæ Venetæ one pound, let these boile againe at a gentle fire till the wine be consumed: then take it off and straine it againe, and so reserue it to your vse. This balme, as it is héere published, is supposed not to be inferior to any balme, be it Indian balme or other: therefore I would not haue men to adde, or take fro, any thing in this balme contained. For what doth it profit them, to go about to better the thing, which of it selfe is already perfectly good, and thus I conclude. The vertues will praise themselues, wherefore it is néedlesse to vse any farther spéeches and circumstances héerein, onely this one briefe note among many I will declare. It happened in *Anno* 1575. a Barber Surgeon, whose name is called *William Clarke* dwelling in Southwarke, hauing in his house a lewd seruant, about the age of 17. or 18. yéeres, wanting the grace of God, did in his masters absence, by the entisement of the diuell, cut his owne throte with a knife, so that part of his drinke, for the space of sixe or seuen daies issued out of the wound. I was presently called to the cure, and first of all I stitched vp the wound, and then I applied thereunto the foresaid balme warme, and staied his bléeding with *Galens* powder, and I very carefully defended the wound from the iniurie of the aire, and so for that present time I ended with conuenient rowling and bolstering. But in such a case there is also required the good helpe of the hand, to kéepe fast and close to the medicines, and all helpes will be little ynough, as I haue well approoued, then after I made ready to vse with the balme, this vnguent called Vnguentum consolidatiuum, and oftentimes also I vsed Vnguentum Nicotian, or De peto.

A briefe note of a yoong man, which with a knife did cut his owne throte.

R. Gummi

℞. Gummi Arab.
Dragagant dissolut. in Aceto } ana. ℥.j.
Sarcocol. ʒ.ij.
Sandarachæ
Hypocistidæ } ana. ʒ.j.
Mastichis
Thuris } ana. ʒ.j.ß.
Tutiæ præparatæ ʒ.j.ß.
Olei Mastichis ℥.iij.
Ceræ q.s.
Misce.

And vpon the same the Gum plaister, and then I applied about the parts néere vnto the wound that defensiue, which is set downe in this booke Cap. 15. Thus he was by me cured, and after sent home to his friends and kinsfolks into the countrie. Yet at the first I was out of all hope or conceit to do him any good, he was so disordered, still pulling off his rowlers and medicines, and faine would haue died, he cared not by what means: till in the end I procured the preacher to be sent for, whose godly perswasions caused him greatly to bewaile and repent his former misdéeds, &c. I could héer nominate other persons so wounded, and by me cured, but for some speciall causes I will leaue them héere vnreuealed or spoken of.

Or this,

A decocted Balme.

℞. Olei comm. lib.iiij.
Terebinthinæ lib.ij.
Aquæ vitæ lib.ij.
Vini odoriferi lib.ij.
Viridis æris in pul. ℥.ij.
Misce.

Boile all these togither according to Art, and last put in your Viridis æris. This was a balme commonly vsed in London in times past amongst the old practisers, &c, who did therewith many excellent cures.

Or this,

A Balme. Am. Pare.

℞. Terebinthinæ Venetæ lib.j.
Gummi Elemni ℥.iiij.
Boli Armeniaci
Sanguinis draconis } ana. ℥.j.
Olei Hyperici cum gummo ℥.iij.
Aquæ vitæ ℥.ij.

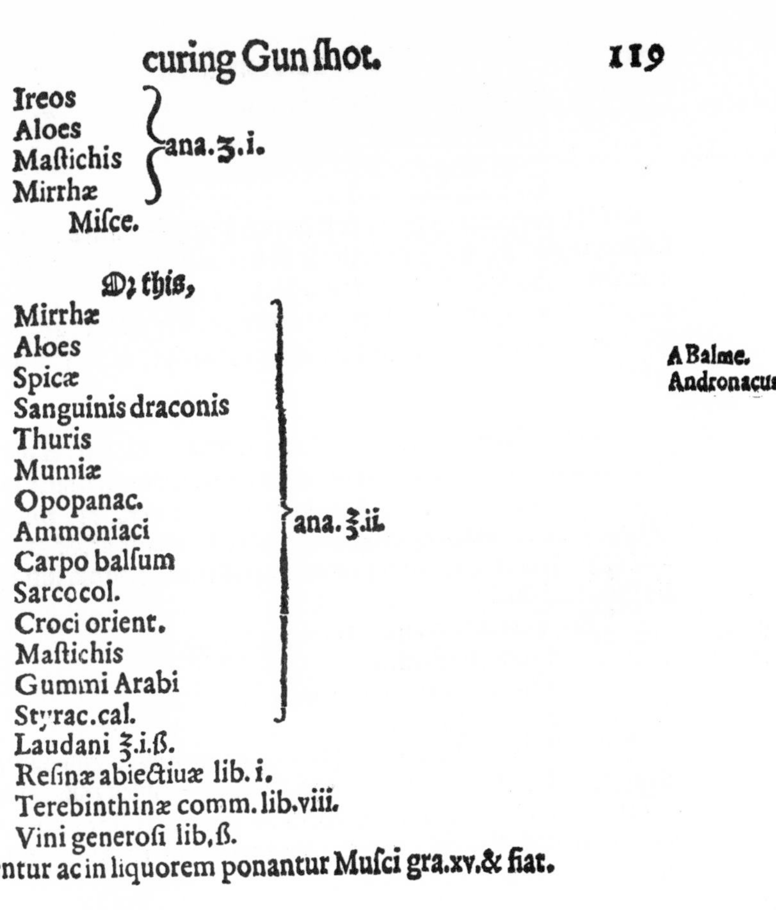

Ireos
Aloes
Mastichis
Mirrhæ
ana.ʒ.i.
Misce.

Or this,

Mirrhæ
Aloes
Spicæ
Sanguinis draconis
Thuris
Mumiæ
Opopanac.
Ammoniaci
Carpo balsum
Sarcocol.
Croci orient.
Mastichis
Gummi Arabi
Styrac.cal.
ana.℥.ii.
Laudani ℥.i.ß.
Resinæ abiectiuæ lib.i.
Terebinthinæ comm. lib.viii.
Vini generosi lib.ß.

A Balme. Andronacus.

Distillentur ac in liquorem ponantur Musci gra.xv.& fiat.

Or this,

℞. Terebinthinæ lib.i.
Olibani ℥.ii.
Aloes succotrinæ
Gariophyllorum
Galing.
Cinnamomi
Croci
Nucis muscatæ
Cubebarum
ana.℥.i.

A very good Balme.

Distill these according to Art, &c.

Or this,

℞. Olei Terebinthinæ lib.i.

Vitellorum

A Balme or oile. Maſter Keble.

Vitellorum ouorum ℥.xiiii.
Reſinæ pini } ana.℥.iii.
Myrrhæ
Gummi hederæ ℥.ii.

Let the yelkes of egges be firſt ſodden hard, then mixe al togither in a ſtillitorie, and with a ſoft fire, let it be drawne, and there will come firſt a water, and laſt the oile, the which yee ſhall reſerue: for it healeth wounds very ſpeedily. This oile was greatly eſteemed of my maſter M. *George Keble*, but whether he were the author of it, I do not certainly know.

Glanfields Balme for wounds made with gun ſhot, &c. A man greatly honored, amongſt warlike men, who alwaies did attribute to him, the title he iuſtly deſerued: To be a man of great induſtry, much practiſe, & experience in Surgery, and ſo cenſured by many other worthy perſons of great account, which were his patients, and did full well know his excellent ſkill.

Glanfields Balme.

℞. Terebinthinę Venetæ } ana. ℥.iiii.
Gummi Elemni
Olei lumbricorum lib.ß.
Aquæ vitæ ℥.j.

Boile theſe, till all the Aqua vitæ be conſumed and waſted cleane away, then take it from the fire and ſtraine it: which done, ad to it Aloes Epaticæ, and of Cinabrii, both made into a very fine powder, ana.ʒi. and put it vnto the reſt, ſtirring it a little, and then reſerue it to your vſe, &c.

Olei hyperici. Clowes.

Olei Hyperici.

℞. Vini Albi lib.ii.
Olei veteris lib.iiii.
Olei Terebinthinæ lib. ij.
Florum Hyperici recentum q.s.

Let the herbs be well bruſed, and put in a double glaſſe, with the oiles and wine, and ſo ſet this in the ſun ſeauen daies, then boile it ſix or ſeauen houres in Balneo Mariæ, then ſtraine it, and put to the wine and oiles, new freſh flowers and ſeedes, and let it ſtand alſo in the ſun other ſeauen daies, then boile it againe in Balneo Mariæ, thus do, ſo many times till the oile be red, and that the wine be conſumed, then ſtraine it, and adde thereto,

Aloes hepaticæ } ana. ℥.i.
Myrrhæ
Maſtichis

Mummiæ

Mummiæ, }
Olibani } ana. ℥. j.
Gariophyllorum }
Macis }
Nucis muscatæ } ana. ℥. ß.
Cinnamomi }
Croci ʒ. i.
Granorum tinctorum ana. ℥. ß.
Vermium terrestrium ℥. iiii.

Let the wormes be purely purged and clensed in Vini albi, q. s. Then put all togither in a double glasse to the oile, and set it in the sun a month, and last of all, let it be boiled againe in Balneo Mariæ twelue houres, being very close stopped, then take it off the fire, and let it rest til it be néere colde, and straine it, and so reserue it to your vse. This oile, I oftentimes vse in the stéed of my balme, and it is also good for the palsey, cramps, aches, and likewise for wounds and pricks in the sinewes, and also for poisoned wounds. And whereas some suppose, that earth wormes be not profitable in this oile, or such like, I can not but thinke their experience very little, and their iudgement much lesse herein.

Mel rosatum.

℞. Of red Rose leaues before they be blowne, two pound, stampe them, and let them be boiled in Aqua cælesti fower pound: after let them be strongly strained, which done, adde thereto of the iuice of red roses well purified, fower pound, and of clarified hony fower pound: let them boile according to Art. Note that your rose leaues and water rest infused togither six or seauen daies before you boile them, as aforesaid. Some in the stéed of Aquæ cælestis, put in wine, and hold it better for some causes, &c. Mel rosatum. Wecker.

A playster very good for gréene wounds, practised in the Lowe Countries, by master *Ierom Farmer*, a Gentleman greatly addicted to Chirurgery, who gaue it me for one of *Paracelsus* plaisters, but in which of *Paracelsus* bookes he had this plaister, I do not certainly know. Paracelsus plaister so called by master Ierom Farmer.

℞. Rad. consolidæ maioris lib. j.
Fol. Ophioglossi lib. j. ß.
Vermium terrest. lib. ß.
Aristolochiæ rotundæ recent. ℥. i.

All these being gréene, beate them well, and then adde to Vini albi, ſo much in quantity as will couer all theſe herbes, ſéeth them in a double veſſell well nealed ten houres: theſe being then ſtrained and taken out, put in new herbes and rootes, and boile it as aforeſaid, and then put to it Butyri recentis q.s. All theſe being mixed togither, let it be boiled in a double veſſell, which being effectually done, then ſtraine it, and after ſet it in the ſun, and reſerue it to your vſe. Then take of the foreſaid oile, and Virgine wax, of ech a pound and a halfe, of Lithargyrij lib.i. Plumbi vſti loti lib. ß. Terebinthinæ ℥.iiii. Ammoniaci, Bdellii ana. ℥. ß. Galbani Opopanacis ana. ʒ.vi. Infuſe theſe gums in viniger, and ſo make a plaiſter according to Art. This plaiſter was giuen me by the gentleman aboue named, when I was in Arnam, at that time when Nemigham was beſieged by the Earle of Leiceſter, &c. I ſay, he deſired me to put it in practiſe, at which time, diuers of our men were wounded and hurt, as well with ſhot as otherwiſe: It hapned, a horſeman was wounded néere the middle of his right thigh, and ſo paſſed vpwards, and by good fortune, it reſted vpon Os pubis, otherwiſe he had béen ſlaine: neuertheleſſe, he was greatly féebled, by reaſon of extreme bléeding. So happily, I hauing things about me, ſtaied his flux of blood: at the next dreſſing I applied a defenſiue about the wound, and then I warmed ſome of the oile of Hypericon, mentioned before in this booke, the which I ſiringed, or iniected into the bottom of the wound, then I made a very ſhort tent, whereon I applied Vnguentum de Peto, or Nicotian, and vpon the ſame, the foreſaid plaiſter. Thus I dreſſed him fiue or ſix daies togither, and then I left out the tent, and with the application of the plaiſter he was cured in fourtéene daies, and ſo ready to ſerue in field againe.

A horſeman wounded with a pike.

Or this,

Emplaſtrum ſticticum.

℞. Ceræ nouæ lib. ß.
Olei oliuarum lib.ij.
Lithargyrii triti lib. i. ß.
Galbani, Opopanacis } ana. ℥.ii.
Ammoniaci, Bdellij } ana. ℥.iii.
Ariſtolochiæ vtriuſque, Calaminaris, Mirrhæ, Thuris } ana. ℥.
Terebinthinæ puræ ℥.iiii.
Miſce.

This

This plaister is to be made with great Art and cunning, the gums must be dissolued in good wine viniger fower and twenty howers, and after boiled, till the viniger be euaporated, then it must be strongly strained, and in the boiling of the said plaister, the gums must be put in by little and little, alwaies stirring them till the gums be incorporated with the rest, last put in your Terebinthin, and so make a plaister according to Art.

Or this,

Another plaister called also Emplastrum sticticum.

℞. Ceræ lib.i.
Colophoniæ ℥.iiii.
Corneoli.
Corallorum rub. & alborum, Lapidis magnetis, Calaminaris } ana. ℥.ß.
Carabis, Mastichis, Thuris } ana. ʒ. vi.
Mirrhæ, Mumiæ } ana.℥.i.ß.
Terebinthinæ ℥.i.ß.
Misce.

Let your waxe and Colophone be relented ouer a gentle fire of coles, then straine it, and adde to the foresaid powders, being very finely powdered and searsed, stirring it continually, and when it is brought to a perfect body, last of all put in your Terebinthinæ, and so make it vp accordingly, &c.

The gum plaister good for wounds made with Gun shot, &c.

The gum plaister.

℞. Axungiæ porcinæ lib.iii.
Olei veteris lib.ii.
Radicum Bryoniæ & Altheæ } ana.lib.ß.

Let these stande infused ten daies, then put all into the pan, and boile them togither ouer a soft fire one houre, then straine them, and ad to the straining,

Lythargyrii auri læuigati lib.iii.
Vitrioli ℥.iiii.

Boile all these togither, til they come to the forme of a sirup, and ad vnto it,

Gummi opopanacis } ana. lib.i.
Ammoniacæ

Dissolue your gums in good wine viniger, which done, then boile all togither againe on a gentle fire of coles, continually stirring them, vntill they be brought to the forme of a plaister, & then when it is neere colde, make it vp in rowles. This plaister is very good to resolue and appease pains, and it is well approued for wounds made with gun shot, and many other excellent vertues it hath, which I haue manifested in many places of this booke, &c.

A plaister of gum Elemni, for wounds in the head. Arceus.

A plaister of gum Elemni for wounds in the head.

℞. Gummi elemni ℥.iii.
Resinæ pini purissimæ
Gummi Ammoniaci
Gummi hederæ
Ceræ } ana. ℥.ii.
Terebinthinæ ℥.iii. ß.
Olei ros. ℥.i. ß.

Let all these boile togither, except the gum Ammoniack, with one cup and a halfe of odoriferous wine, vnto the consumption thereof, adde in the end the Ammoniack dissolued in viniger, and your gum Hederæ finely powdred, & being sufficiently boiled, let it be wrought vp in wine and Aqua vitæ, and so make it vp in rowles, &c.

A plaister which is called Flos vnguentorum.

Emplastrum quod dicitur, Flos vnguentorum.

℞. Resinæ
Resinæ pini } ana. ℥.viij.
Ceræ albæ
Olibani } ana. ℥.iiij.
Mastichis &
Mirrhæ } ana. ℥.i.
Adipis ceruini ℥.iiii.
Camphor. ʒ.ii.
Vini albi lib.iiii.
Terebinthinæ ℥.iii.

Misce & fiat emplastrum secundum artem.

Emplastrum diachalcitheos.

Emplastrum diachalcitheos,

℞. Olei vet. lib.iii.
Axungiæ vet. sine sale lib.ii.
Lithargyrii triti lib.iii.
Vitrioli ℥.iiij.

Let

Let your litharge (saith my Author) be steeped twelue howers in the oile to boile, then to a iust thicknes, putting in the Axungiæ, stirring it cōtinually with a Spatula, either of the Date trée, or of the Oke trée: whē it is boiled ynough, take all from the fire, and put in your Vitrioll, being first beatē into fine powder, &c. Friendly reader, for that diuers men are very desirous to make this plaister very white in colour, and yet haue for the most part mist of their purpose, but haue made it sometimes of one colour, & somtimes of another: therefore to satisfie such men, howsoeuer I estéeme not of the colour, so it work the true effect yet: I haue obtained of a friend ỹ way to make it very white. He did take thrée pounds of litharge of gold as aforesaid, being powdered & searsed through a fine cloth, then take so much in waight of white salt being in powder, and mingle it with the litharge, & let it stand one day and a night: then put to the litharge & salt: so much water that it doth swim ouer the litharge thrée fingers, & let it stand eight dais, stirring it six or seuen times a day, & let it remaine so vntill all be perfect white, and being white put in a great deale of water to it, and stir it well, and let it settle one day: then put away that water, and so refresh it, vntill you taste no saltnes in the water: and thus the litharge will be very white, and then make your plaister with a soft fire, without flame or smoke, as you are vsed to do in others, &c.

A way to make this plaister very white.

The white Mucilage plaister,

The white Mussilage plaister.

℞. Cerusæ lib.v.
Lithargyrii auri lib.ii.
Olei comm. lib.viii.
The rootes of marsh Mallowes being cleansed and picked from the pith m.iiii.
Seminis Lini & Fœnigræci contus. ana.m.i.
Water q.s. and make héereof the Mucilage, whereof take lib.iii.
Misce, & fiat emplastrum secundum artem.

A resolutiue plaister very good in cold and windie swellings, and is commonly called the Cummin plaister,

The Cummin plaister.

℞. Olei Anethini lib.ß.
Resinæ lib.iii.
Resinæ pini lib.ii.
Ceræ citrinæ lib.i.
Pulueris baccarum Lauri } ana. lib.i.
& Seminis Cummini }

Let

Let the sædes be made into very fine powder as possibly may be, but first relent your Perrosin rosin and ware togither, and so straine it, then by little and little strow in your powders, and in the end, when it wareth somwhat colde, with spæde make it vp in rowles, working in the oyle with your hands, and so reserue it to your vse, &c.

A Sparadrop plaister,

A Sparadrop plaister. M.Keble.

℞. Olei comm. lib. ii.
Plumbi albi & Plumbi rubi } ana. ℥. xi.
Ceræ ℥. vi.

Boile all these togither, till it ware blacke, and in the coling put in

Adipis anatis & caponis } ana. ℥. i.
Camphoræ ℥. ß.
Misce.

Fréndly Reader, I haue as much as in me lieth, in diuers places of this boke, truly commended the worthines and dignitie of euery good mans knowledge and skill, neither haue I vnaduisedly discommended any, but such as deserue the ill opinion of the world, and according to their due, I haue rightly spoken of them: moreouer, I must néedes say, Master *Banister* for his knowledge and iudgement in the Art, and for publishing of certaine bokes of Surgerie in the English tong, for the good of our countrie and common wealth, deserueth double honor and praise of all men.

A plaister to be vsed for drie stitches in wounds of the face, &c, I do vse to take one ounce of this plaister, and one ounce of Emplastrum contra rupturam, and it is the better for this purpose.

A plaister for dry stitches in the face, &c. I.B.

℞. Resinæ
Resinæ pini
Picis nigri } ana. ℥. iiii.
Mastichis
Mirrhæ
Thuris
Olibani
Aloes hepat.
Terebinthinæ } ana. ℥. i.
Gummi Dragagant. ℥. vi.
Misce.

A Plaister which master *Francis Rassius* Chirurgeon to the French king did giue vnto me, for one of his best secrets, and it is chiefly vsed to

kéepe

keepe open issues, as my selfe with him haue seene the experience of it vpon persons of great account.

A plaister to keepe open any issue. Franciscus Rassius.

℞. Ceræ albæ lib.ß.
Viridis æris ℥.iii.
Mercurii sublimati ℥.i.
Misce.

Heere follow certaine needfull and necessarie vnguents for wounds made with Gun shot, &c.

Two proper and peculiar medicines, which are good to stay the gleeting Mucilage humour of wounds in the ioints, often practised by master *Balthrop* late Sergeant Surgeon vnto hir Maiestie, being a man of a rare and exquisite experience in Chirurgerie: one in whom the olde prouerbe might very well be verified, that is, To haue a Lions hart, a Ladies hand, and a Haukes eie, and what else is required in a good Surgeon was truly found in him.

Vnguentum Resinæ. Sergeant Balthrop.

℞. Resinæ ℥.v.
Terebinthinæ ℥.viii.
Mellis lib.i.
Mirrhæ } ana.℥.i.
Sarcocollæ }
The Mucilages of Fenigreeke and of Lineseede, being made with white wine ana.℥.j.

Mixe these togither, and make heereof an vnguent according to art. To the same intent and purpose this vnguent following was by him greatly commended,

℞. Mirrhæ, and Aquæ vitæ, of each equall portions, grinde them togither vpon a painters stone, that is pure and cleane, and labour them so long till they come to the forme of an vnguent, &c.

A good mundifieng vnguent called Lipsius, vsed in the Hospital of S. Bartholomew, by men of great experience in the Art of Surgery, specially for vlcers in the mouth, &c.

Vnguentum Lipsium, a very good Mundificatiue.

℞. Mellis com.lib.ii.
Vitrioli albi ℥.iiii.
Succi Caprifolii lib.iiii.

First boile the iuice and the Mel togither till it come to the thicknes of hony, and last put in your Vitrioll and boile it a little: and so reserue it to your vse, &c.

An

A linament which doth mundifie and incarne wounds in the head. Arceus.

An vnguent or liniment which doth mundifie and incarne wounds in the head.

℞. Terebinthinæ claræ }
Gummi elemni } ana.℥.i.ß.
Pinguedinis castoratæ ℥.ii.
Pinguedinis porcinæ antiquæ ℥.i.
Misce & fiat vnguentum.

A good mundifieng vnguent called also Vnguentum viride.

Vnguentum Mundificatiuum, **called also** Vnguentum viride.

℞. Resinæ }
Resinæ pini } ana.lib.i.
Ceræ citrinæ }
Olei com. lib.ii.
Terebinthinæ lib.i.
Viridis æris ℥.i.
Misce & fiat vnguentum.

Vnguentum incarnatiuum regis Angliæ.

Vnguentum incarnatiuum regis Angliæ.

℞. Ceræ albæ }
Resinæ } ana.℥.iiii.
Terebinthinæ ℥.i.
Thuris }
Mastichis } ana.℥.ß.
Olei com. ℥.iii.
Misce & fiat Vnguentum.

Vnguentum incarnatiuum M. Keble.

Vnguentum incarnatiuum magistri Keble.

℞. Resinæ }
Ceræ } ana.℥.iiii.
Terebinthinæ ℥.ii.
Olei com ℥.viii.
Mellis ℥.iii.
Vitellorum ouorum numero iiii.
Misce & fiat vnguentum.

Vnguentum incarnatiuum Clowes.

Vnguentum incarnatiuum.

℞. Ceræ Citrinæ lib.ß.
Resinæ ℥.vi.
Terebinthinæ ℥.v.
Olei rosarum lib.ß.

Mastichis

Maſtichis
Olibani
Mirrhæ
Sarcocollæ } ana.℥.ß.
Aloes ʒ.ii.
Croci ʒ.i.
Mellis roſ.℥.iiii.
Miſce & fiat vnguentum.

Vnguentum Baſilicon.

Vnguentum baſilicon.

℞. Reſinæ
Terebinthinæ
Adipis vaccini
Picis naualis } ana. lib.j.
Olei comm. lib.iii.
Ceræ lib.ii.
Miſce & fiat vnguentum.

Some haue altered the doſes héerof into leſſe quantities, and then adde to it Olibanum as followeth, and call it Vnguentum Macedonium, and it is indéed for ſome cauſes greatly bettered.

℞. Reſinæ
Picis nigræ
Adipis vaccini
Terebinthinæ
Olibani } ana.℥.ii.
Olei ℥.vi.
Ceræ ℥.iiii.
Fiat Vnguentum.

Vnguentum Sanatiuum.

Vnguentum ſanatiuum.

℞. Lapidis calaminaris præparati ℥.iiii.
Ceruſæ lotæ in aqua roſ. ℥.j.
Lithargyrij auri loti ℥.ii.
Olei roſ. lib.ß.
Seui ouini ℥.ij.
Terebinthinæ lotæ in aqua roſ. ℥.ij.ß.
Ceræ citr. q.s.
Camphoræ ʒ.j.
Miſce & fiat vnguentum.

R Vnguentum

Vnguentum pro Spasmo.

Vnguentum pro Spasmo.

℞. Axungiæ cerui, Taxi, Vrci, ana. ℥.i.
Olei laurini ℥.i.ß.
Olei vulpini, Castorei, Terebinthinæ, Iuniperi, Lumbrici, ana. ℥.ß.
Vnguenti Agrippæ & Dialthæ, ana. ℥.ii.

Let the Terebinthinæ be washed in the water of Lillies, then take,
Euphorbii. ℈.i.
Cum modica cera.
Misce & fiat Vnguentum.

An vnguent commonly called, Vnguentum neruale, or Oleum Neruorum. I haue many times seene this oile vsed with great profit to the patient, and for that I neuer read it in any english author, I haue therefore thought it good here to publish the same for the benefit of others, &c.

Oleum Neruorum.

℞. Eupatorii, Camomillæ, Betonicæ, Saluiæ, Menthæ, Hederæ terrestris, Abrotani, Arthemisiæ, Absinthii, Nasturtii, Maluarum, Origani, Pulegii, Auriculæ muris, Solani, Chamæpityos, Vrticæ, Fol. lauri, Ebulii, Costi, ana. ℥.iii.

Serpentariæ

Serpentariæ
Enulæ camp.
Rubiæ maioris
Herbæ paralyſis
Rutæ
Raphani
Sambucæ
Ariſtolochiæ longæ } ana. ℥.iij.
Apii
Rad. altheæ
Cyclamini
Calendulæ
Caulis rub.
Calaminthæ
Centaurii minoris
Vitis albæ
Hyperici
Butyri Maialis lib.xii.
Ceræ virgineæ lib. i.
Seui arietis ℥. xii.
Axungiæ gallinæ ℥.vi.
Axungiæ anſeris ℥. iii.
Olibani ℥.xii.
Olei laurini lib.viii.
Miſce ſecundum artem.

A liniment for windy tumors.

A liniment for windy tumors.

℞. Oleorum chamæmeli
Anethi } ana. ℥. ii.
Lauri
Ceræ albæ } ana.q.s.
Aquę vitæ
Miſce.

A moſt excellent remedy for the curing of cold, hard, and windie ſwellings in the armes and legs, being well approued by a very ſkilfull Phyſition in this citie of London, which ſecret he deliuered vnto me, as it is here deſcribed, H. O.

A ſpeciall remedy for cold, hard, and windy ſwellings. H.O.

℞. Saponis nigri
Axungiæ porcinæ } ana. lib. i.
Aquæ vitæ
Miſce.

You must first relent your Axungiæ and Saponis togither, then put thereto the one halfe of the Aqua vitæ, and boile it till the Aqua vitæ be euaporated away: after put thereunto the rest of the Aqua vitæ, and boile it gently as before said, which done, reserue it to your vse, &c.

A linament to cease pain, and cause sleepe.

A liniment to cease paine, and cause sléepe, being applied vnto the temples.

R. Opii extracti cum aceto ros. ℥. i.
Sem. Hyoscyami albi ʒ.vj.
Nucis musc. ʒ. v.
Vnguenti ros. ℥.ii. ß.
Olei nucis musc. gut.
Fiat linimentum.

An vnguent very good to cure inflammations.

An Vnguent very good for inflammations.

R. Vnguenti populeonis, Vnguenti ros. } ana. ℥. ß.

Let these be well washed first in rose water, and last in plantine water q.s. adding thereto
Olei ros. ℥.iiii.
Cerusæ ℥.ii.
Ceræ albæ q.s.
Terræ sigillatæ ℥.i.ß.
Camphoræ ℈. ii.
Opii ℈. i.
Misce & fiat vnguentum.

Vnguentum populeum, Nicolai & Weckeri.

Vnguentum populeum *Nicolai & Weckeri*.

R. The buds of Poplar being gréene and picked very cleane, lib. j. ß. Axungiæ porcinæ lib. iiii. the poplar buds must be bruised & mixed with the Axungiæ, vntill your other herbs may be prepared, then adde to it

Fol. papaueris agrestis
Fol. mandragoræ
Fol. Hyosciami
Solani
Vermicularis aut crassulæ
Lactucæ
Semperuiui
Bardanæ
Portulacæ
} ana. ℥. iii.

Florum

Florum violarum
Vmbilici Veneris
Summitatum pruni tenerarum } ana. ℥.iij.

These herbs must be mixed and tempered with Axungiæ as aforesaid, then adde thereto Vini optimi, quantum satis est. Boile these to the consumption of the wine, then straine them, and make an vnguent according to Art. It is very good against extreme raging heats & feuers, it prouoketh sleepe, the temples being therewith annointed, &c.

Vnguentum infrigidans *Galeni*.

Vnguentum infrigidans Galeni.

℞. Olei ros. ℥.iii.
Ceræ albæ ℥.ß.

Melt these togither, and being well washed with rose viniger and rose water, reserue it to your vse, &c.

Vnguentum album *Rhazis*.

Vnguentum album Rhazis.

℞. Olei com. lib.ii.
Cerus. subtilissimæ lib.j.
Ceræ albæ ℥.vj.
Camphoræ ʒ.ii.

Your oile and waxe must be relented togither on a gentle fire of coles, and when it waxeth neere cold, strow in your ceruse, and last of all put in your Camphor dissolued in oile of roses, &c.

A singular good vnguent called Vnguentum nutritum, very profitable for all inflammations, practised by Master *Godorus* Sergeant Surgeon vnto hir Maiestie: the which said vnguent I haue seene him vse to his great credit, and he gaue the said vnguent vnto me, with diuers other worthy secrets, a most sufficient assurance of his kindnes and good will, and an euident testimonie of his brotherly loue and vnfained friendship, which no doubt ought to be betweene euery good friend and friend, specially being all of one fellowship, art, and profession, then neede not we care for the flattering intruder, neither the glosing vnderminer, or such like wicked sowers of sedition, which kinde of men, to auoid suspition of their wicked dealings, vse a pretie kind of cunning in the couering of such coloured practises, vnder many false, flattering, and fained faire words.

Vnguentum nutritum. Sergeant Godorus.

℞. Lithargyrij auri ℥.iiii.
Olei comm. lib.j.

Aceti

Aceti vini albi distillati ℥.viij.

Misce,& fiat vnguentum secundum artem.

A Cataplasma for brused wounds.

A Cataplasma for brused wounds.

℞. Rad.Altheæ lib.ß.
Fol.Mal.& Violar. ana.m.j.

Terantur,coquantur,& exprimantur,deinde adde

Butyri &
Olei comm. } ana.℥.iij.
Vitellorum ouorum numero iij.
Croci, modicum.
Farinæ triticeæ &
Hordei q.s.

Fiat Cataplasma.

A very good Cataplasma for the cure of Gangræna.

A Cataplasma very good for the cure of Gangræna.

℞. Far.fab.
Hordei
Orobi
Lupin. } ana.lib.ß.
Salis comm.
Mellis ros. } ana.℥.iiij.
Succi Absinthij
Marrub. } ana.℥.ij.ß.
Aloes
Mirrhæ,&
Aquæ vitæ } ana.℥.ij.
Oximel simp. q.s.

Misce,& fiat Cataplasma.

A Cataplasma for windie tumours or swellings.

A Cataplasma for windy tumors or swellings.

℞. Fol.Chamæmeli
Meliloti
Anethi
Ros.rub.pul. } ana.m.j.
Foliorum Mal.&
Absinthij } ana.m.ß.
Furfuris m.j.

Boile

Boile all theſe togither in Lixiuio,& vino rub. then adde thereto

Medullæ panis }
Farinæ fab. } ana.q.s.
Olei roſ.& }
Mirtini } ana.℥.ij.
Miſce.

Galens Reſtrictiue powder.

Galens powder to ſtay great fluxes of blood.

℞. Olibani ℥.ij.
Aloes hepaticæ ℥.j.
Pilorum leporis terrefact. }
& ouorum album. } ana.q.s.
Miſce.

Gales powder for reſtraining great fluxes of blood.

Gales powder to ſtay great fluxes of blood.

℞. Aluminis Succorini }
Thuris }
Arcenici } ana.℥.ij.
Calcis viui ℥.vj.

Make all theſe in fine powder, and put unto them a pint of ſtrong viniger, and boile them on the fire, ſtirring them continually till the viniger be conſumed, then ſet it in the ſunne, or in an ouen till it be perfectly dried, that you may make it in fine powder, and when you will vſe it, take of this powder ℥.iij. Boli Armoniaci ℥.iij. Pulueris Alchimiſtici ℥.j.Miſce, and when you will vſe it for diſmembring, then take the whites of egs alſo q.s.&c. You ought (I ſay) to haue a great and ſpeciall foreſight vnto the intolerable paines and accidents, which are ſtirred vp by reaſon and means of this powder,&c.

Calmetheus Reſtrictiue powder.

Calmetheus powder to ſtay great fluxes of blood.

℞. Boli Armeniaci ℥.vj.
Terræ ſigillatæ ℥.ij.
Farinæ volatilis ℥.ij.
Gypſi }
Calcis vini } ana.℥.iiij.

And when you will vſe of this powder, mixe therewith
Albuminum ouorum q.s.

Puluis sine pare, very good to take away corrupt and spungious flesh.

Puluis siue Pare. Ioan. Arden.

℞. Viridis æris
Auri pigmenti } ana. ℥. ij.
Vitrioli combusti ℥. iiii.
Aluminis combusti ℥. viii.
Et fiat puluis.

The true maner and order of making Mercurii præcipitati. A. P.

The true maner and order of making Mercurii præcipitati. A.P.

℞. Argenti viui lib. ß.
Aqua fortis lib. j.

Put them in a double violl, and make therof a powder as followeth, take a large earthen vessell, wherinto set the forenamed violl that hath the quick siluer and the Aqua fortis in it, strawing ashes vnder it, and so couering it therewith vp to the neck, then put burning coles vnder and about the earthen vessell, so that the Aqua fortis may boile and euaporate forth, and the glasse that containeth it may be without danger of breaking: when all the water is euaporated and fumed forth, which you may knowe when you see no more of the smoke to come forth at the mouth of the glasse, then take it out of the ashes, and in the bottom there you shall find the Mercury calcinated of the colour of red Lead, separated from euery white, yellow, or blacke excrement, that which is congealed white in the top, is called Sublimat, which if it remaine with the lime of the Mercury, it causeth it to be painful: therefore you must separate this Mercury powder by it selfe, & so beat it into powder, and set it ouer the quick coles in a vessel of brasse, stirring it still for the space of an hower or two, for so it will lose a great part of his sharpnes and biting: and therefore it will be lesse painfull when it is applied, &c.

A very good Lixiuium to stay Gangræna comming of a cold cause, by lying in the frost or snow, or the like occasions, wherby the vitall spirits are prohibited to come vnto the mortified part.

A Lixinium for Gangræna comming of a cold cause. M. Keble.

℞. Lixiuii lib. viii.
Lupinorum contusorum ℥. vj.
Orobi ℥. ii.
Salis com. m. j. ß.

Absinthii

Absinthii }
Centaurii } ana.m.i.
Marubii }
Florum Chamæmeli m.j.ß.
Aquę vitæ lib.i.

Boile all these togither till one part be consumed, and so let it rest, and reserue it to your vse, &c.

Another.

Paracelsus.

℞. Piperis longi }
Cardimonii } ana.ʒ.i.
Granorum paradisi }
Euphorbii ʒ.ii.
Mastichis ʒ.i.ß.

Reduce them into powder, and boile them all in two measures of the vrine of a boy, vntill the eight part remain, then straine them, and with that which is left, let the mortified member be annointed or bathed euery day thrise: this will make separation of the quick from the mortified parts aliue. Giue the patient to drinke Ginger, Cloues, Cardamomum, Granum paradisi, &c. boiled in wine and drinke it hot.

Certaine precepts meet for yoong students in Chirurgerie, gathered chiefly out of Guido Decauliaco by William Clowes.

Precepts for yoong students in Chirurgery.

I Read that Aristotle the wise and graue Philosopher,
Wrote an Epistle, vnto noble king Alexander:
Saying, choose your seruitors, by their good & comly face,
For such men are most meete, to be about your grace.
Of the same opinion, the best learned sure are still,
That the countenance doth bewray the maners good or ill.
Therefore saith Guido, you shall in no wise choose
Any such deformed person, Chirurgery to vse,
But one that is ingenious, and apt for to deuise,
New remedies for new grieues, as daily they do rise.

T With

With a cunning, spéedy, handsome handling of the griefe,
By the third part of Physick, procuring safe reliefe.
The things that a good Surgeon, ought chiefly to know
Are naturall, not naturall, against nature also.
Yet they that haue learning without practise in the Art,
Do oft more hurt, than helpe, vnto the gréeued part.
So pracise without learning, yée ought not to admit,
These two may not be separate, that are so duly knit.
There must be a dexterity, and a finenesse in working,
A quick remembrance, and a ready vnderstanding.
He must be circumspect, and séeke to auoide all slaunder,
Not too couetous for mony, but a reasonable demaunder.
Being good vnto the poore, let the rich pay therefore,
So God will blesse thy doings, and thou shalt haue the more.
He must also be honest, and in liuing very vpright,
To serue the Lord our God, must be his whole delight.
Auoiding of all drunkennesse, and vile riot to detest,
Least he grow fit for nothing, but Bacchus belly feast.
His fingers must be small, and his hands without quaking,
Stedfast to hold without trembling or shaking.
Who worketh vpon mans body, being vnskilful of the same,
Is fitter for the stable, than to cure the sicke or lame.
The patients lawfull secrets, you ought for to conceale,
It is not for a Surgeons credit, things secret to reueale.
Likewise the patient ought to suffer, and duly to obserue
The precepts of his surgeon, frõ the which he may not swarue
Hauing good trust in him, and a sure hope and confidence,
And touching all the cure, yéelding due obedience.
A Surgeon should not take in hand any cure or maladie,
The which is past all helpe, or hope of his recouery.
And he that setteth a day, when his patient shall be cured,
Is but a childish Surgeon, you may be well assured.
Hippocrates in his Aphorisme, as Galen writeth sure,
Saith, foure things are néedfull to euery kinde of cure.
The first, saith he, to God belongeth the chiefest part,

The

The ſecond to the Surgeon,who doth apply the art.
The third vnto the medicine,that is dame Natures friend,
The fourth vnto the patient,with whom I hære will end.
How then may a Surgeon appoint a time, day or houre,
When thrée parts of the cure are quite without his powre.
Al theſe things ſhuld be obſerud by ſurgeons as their vowes:
I wiſh we all could follow this, finis William Clowes.

When valiant Mars,with braue and warlike band,
In foughten field,with ſword and ſhield doth ſtand.
May there be miſt a Surgeon that is good,
To ſalue your wounds,and eke to ſtay your blood?

To cure you ſure he will haue watchfull eie,
And with ſuch wights he meanes to liue and die:
So that againe,you muſt augment his ſtore,
And hauing this, he will requeſt no more.

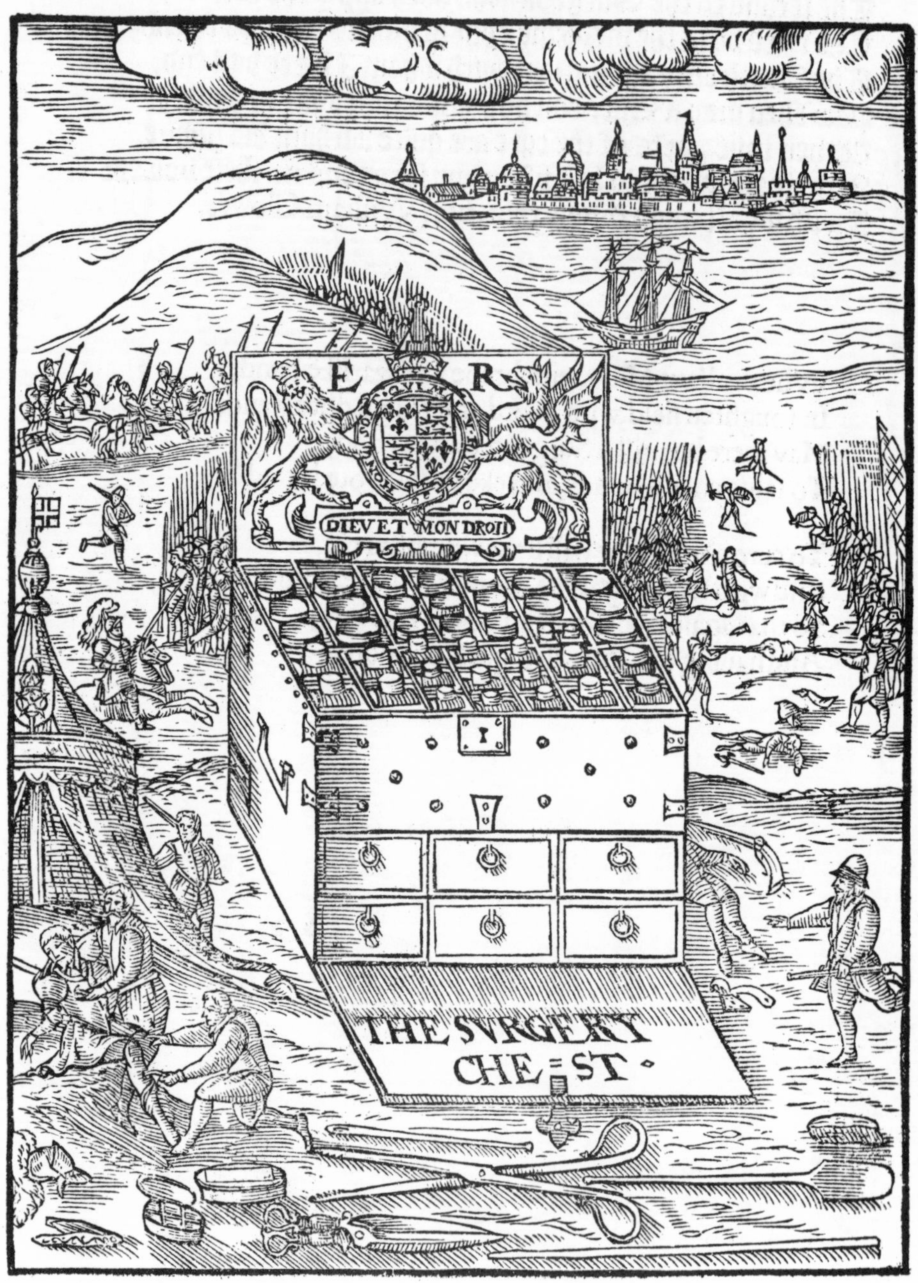
E R
DIEV ET MON DROIT
THE SVRGERY
CHE = ST

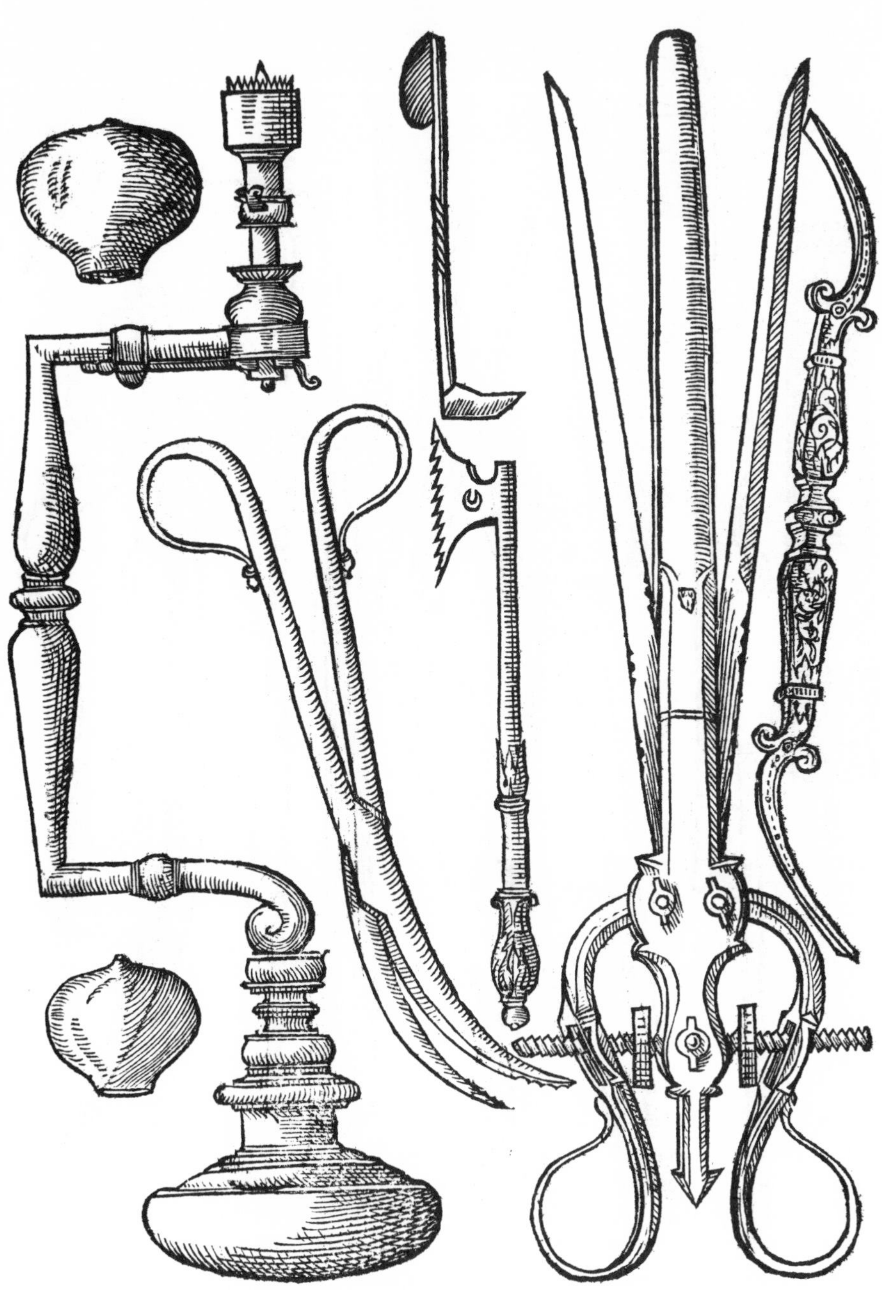

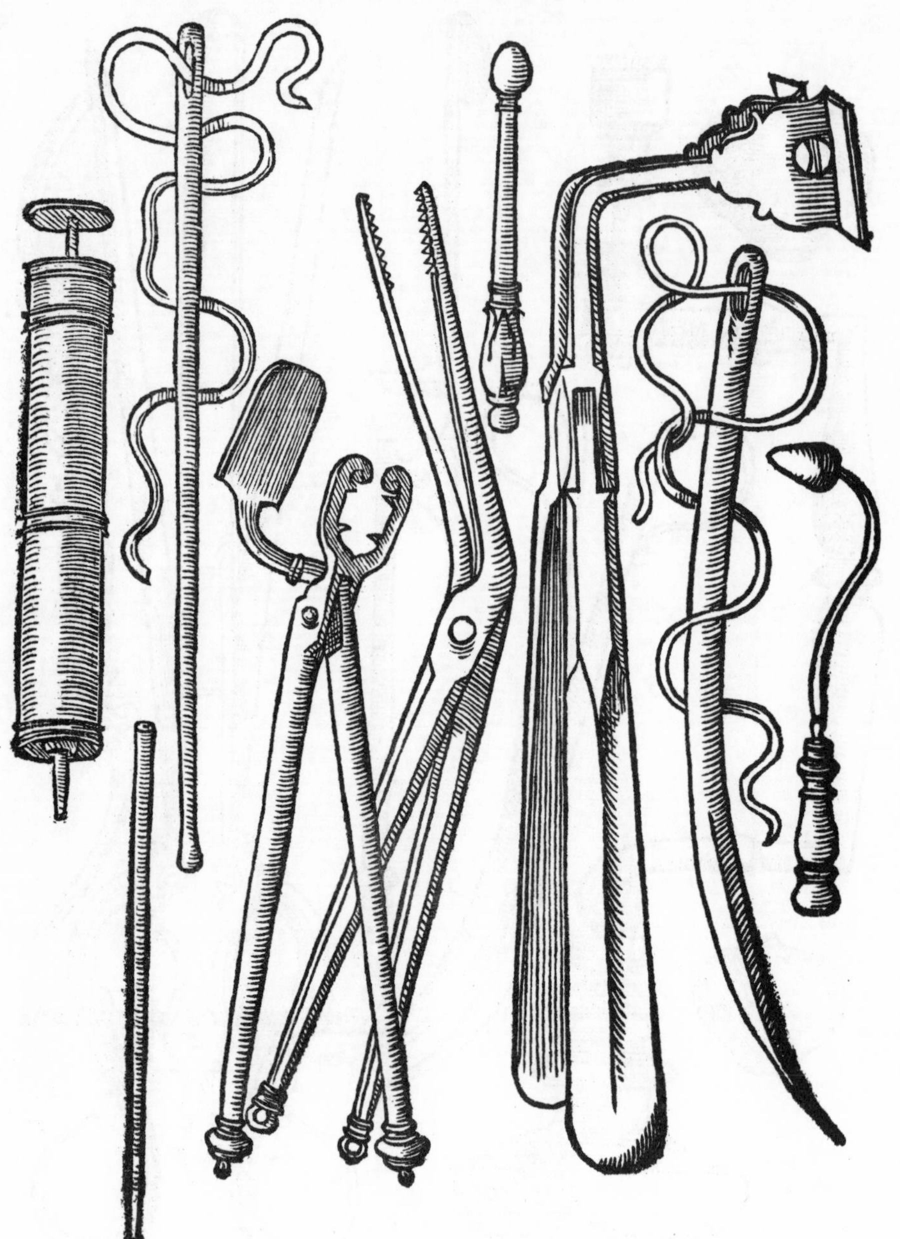

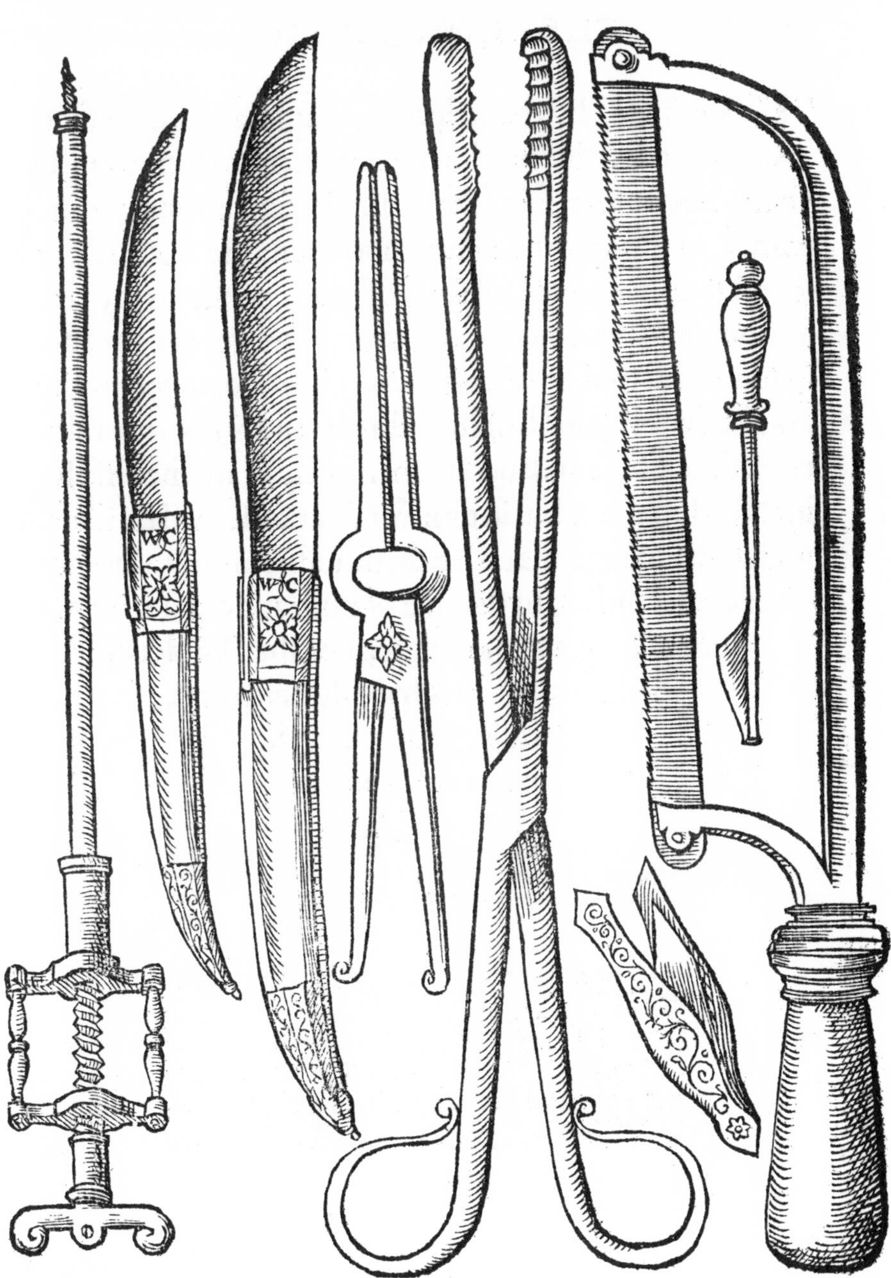
W C
W C

THE CONCLVSION.

THus haue I by the helpe of almightie God, finiſhed and ended this booke of Obſeruations, knowing as I haue heertofore ſaid, that I ſhall make a rude performance of a good meaning : and therefore I aſſure my ſelfe, I ſhall not pleaſe all ſorts of men, neither is it to me any new and vnacquainted matter, to heare that I am deſpiſed and ill ſpoken of, and my works condemned by the abuſe of vnbrideled boldnes : but ſith it argueth the raſhnes of their baſe and inconſtant heads, I care the leſſe for it, and I doubt not but in time for ſhame they wil be ſilent: and in the meane ſpace let them iudge of my dooings heerin, according to the rule of truth and equitie, without cauilling and partialitie, then ſhall I indeede thinke my labours happily beſtowed, and willingly accept an honeſt admonition.

FINIS.

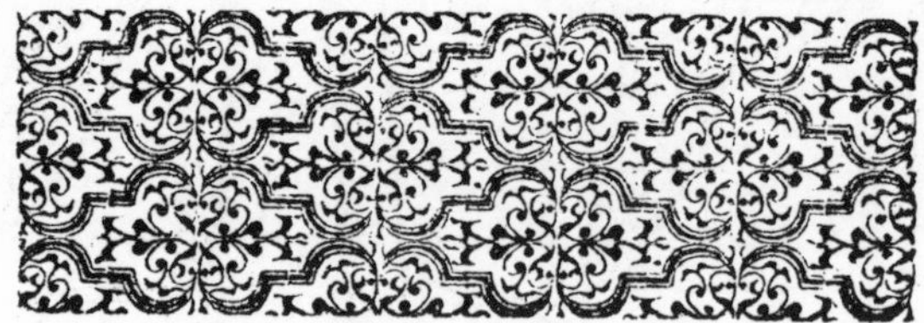

A BRIEFE AND NECESSARY TREATISE, TOVCHING THE CVRE OF THE DISEASE NOW VSVALLY called LVES VENEREA, by vnctions and other approoued waies of curing: newly corrected and augmented in the yeere of our Lord 1596

By WILLIAM CLOWES one of hir Maiesties Chirurgions.

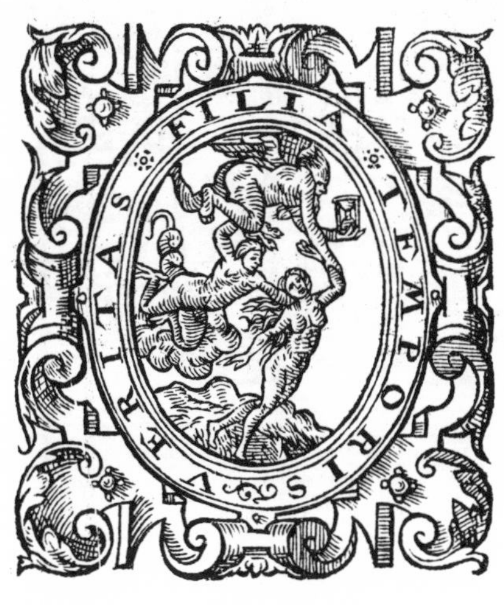

Imprinted at London by Edm. Bollifant, for Thomas Dawson.

1596

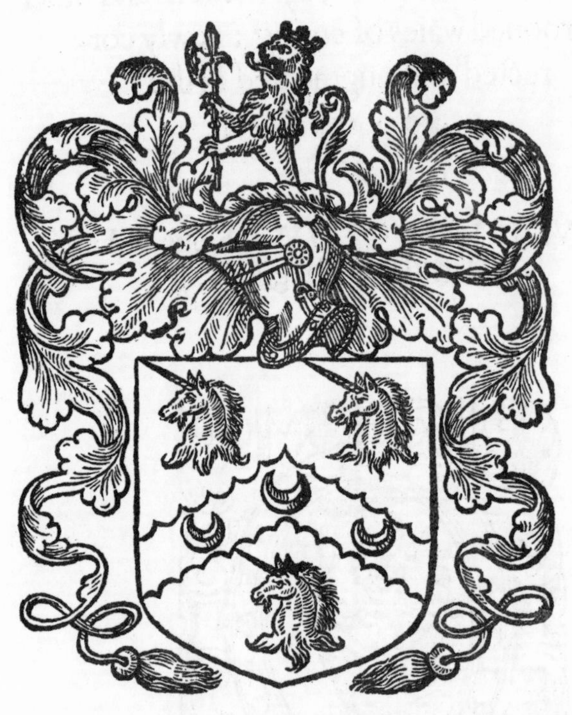

To all yoong professors of Chirurgerie in general, and to the friendly Reader, WILLIAM CLOWES wisheth good health, and all happines in the Lord.

FRiendly Reader, I am at this present to intreate of that disease, and the cure of the same, called in Latine Morbus Gallicus, or Morbus Neapolitanus, but more properly Lues Venerea, a sicknes very lothsome and odious, yea troublesome and dangerous, a notable testimonie of the iust wrath of God against that sinne: which disease aforesaid, I suppose at this day infecteth not onely Naples, Fraunce, and Spaine, but also (as I thinke) it raigneth ouer the face of the whole earth: and therfore is the cure thereof most expedient, profitable, and necessarie to be looked vnto. And as it is a most true saying, that great diseases are not to be cured with great protestation of words, I haue therfore (as much as in me lieth) endeuored my selfe to stop the mouthes of those vile persons, which indeed neuer respect the goodnes of any matter, be it neuer so excellent, but rather seeke with slanderous termes, and false accusations, to finde faults and imperfections with the person of the writer, such is their monsterous ingratitude. Albeit friendly Reader, I must heer confesse, indeed it is not in my learning, power, reason and wit, to write or speake more largely or effectually, for the true cure of this disease, called Lues Venerea, than hath beene already spoken and written of by sundry others far more excellent men before me. Notwithstanding, sith I haue presumed thus farre to write in this short treatise or discourse, of the cure of the foresaid disease, cured by vnctions, very briefly and plainly for the benefit and commoditie of all such as will diligently read, carefully marke, & truly practise the same. Heerin you shall manifestly finde what maner of cure I vsed, and what order of method I followed, with the true vse of all those remedies, the which frõ time to time I administred, in such sort I suppose, that none that carrieth the name of a well minded artist, shall haue iust cause to dislike any thing heerein specified, so shall you receiue also at my hands such other fruits, as I haue heer gathered by mine owne trauell, & also learned of others, and which by practise I haue found to be most certaine & true: therfore I will now proceed no further in discoursing, but briefly giue you to vnderstand, that I was determined to haue written more generally in this treatise, but that I thought it needlesse, sith I vnderstood there was now shortly comming forth a far more learned worke, intreating of the said disease, called Morbus Gallicus, cured also by vnctions, & writtẽ by that great doctor Theredehere of Fraunce, a man of a profound iudgemẽt, and very great experience, as it may appeere by the testimonies of many famous men: which worke of his is now newly translated out of French into English, by M. William Martin Surgeon of London. And so I here conclude with this short preface, crauing friendly acceptance of my harty good wil and faithful zeale vnto my countrie & countrimen, whom I see in these daies exceedingly afflicted with this noisome and perilous sicknes. Farewell.

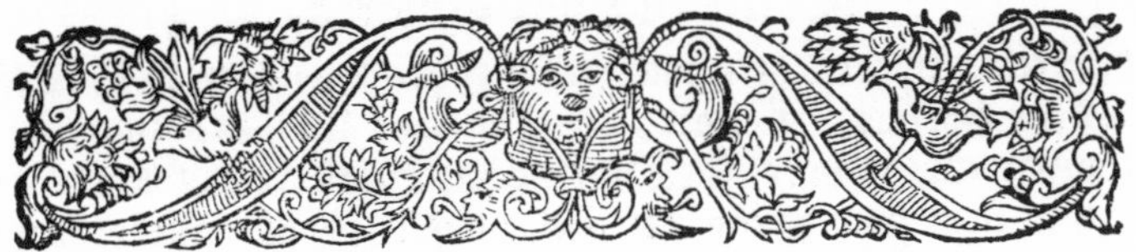

Of the beginning and ſpreading of *Lues Venerea*. Cap.1.

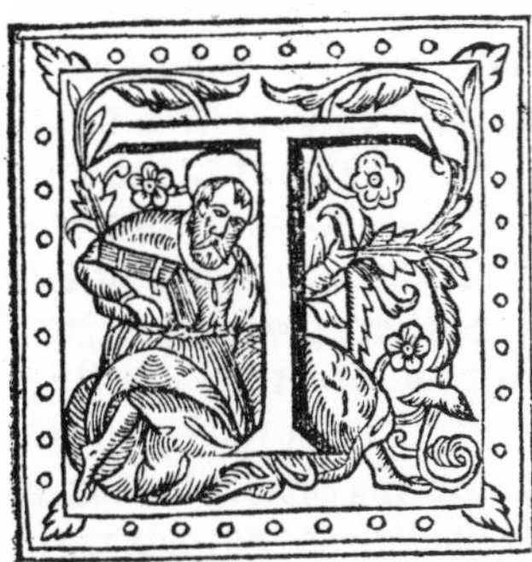

This diſeaſe now vſually called *Lues Venerea*, did firſt appéere, as the learned Phyſitions *Monardus* and *Montanus*, and alſo that learned Surgeon *Vigo*, with others, do affirme, in the yéere of our Lord God, 1494. in the month of December, when the French King tooke his iorney to recouer the kingdom of Naples: at which time hapned amongſt the ſoldiers and people, this diſeaſe to appéere: which was at that time termed by the French men, Morbus Neapolitanus: but they of Naples, called it Morbus Gallicus. Which name, hath ſo in common ſpéech remained with vs vntill this day. I do not héere purpoſe to argue to the contrary, but onely I meane to deliuer vnto you plainly the whole order of the cure, according vnto thoſe gifts and graces, which God of his great goodnes hath beſtowed vpon me.

If I be not deceiued in mine opinion (friendly Reader) I ſuppoſe the diſeaſe it ſelfe was neuer more rife in Naples, Italie, France or Spaine, than it is at this day in the Realme of England. I pray God deliuer vs from it, and to remoue from vs that filthy ſinne that bréedeth it. It is wonderfull to conſider, the huge multitude of ſuch as be infected, and that daily increaſe, to the great danger of many. The cauſes whereof, I ſée none ſo great, as the licentious and beaſtly diſorder of a great number of rogues and vagabonds, the filthy life of many lewde and idle perſons, men and women, about the citie of London, &c. By meanes of which diſordered perſons, ſome other of better diſpoſition are many times infected, and many more like to be, except there be found ſome redreſſe for the ſame: I may ſpeake boldly, bicauſe I ſpeake truly: and yet I do ſpeak it with gréefe of minde, that in the Hoſpitall of Saint Bartholomew in London, there hath béene cured of this diſeaſe by me and thrée others, within fiue yéeres, to the number of one thouſand and more. I ſpeake nothing of Saint Thomas Hoſpitall, and other houſes about

about the citie, wherein an infinite multitude are daily cured. The Maſters of the foreſaid Hoſpitals, being moued with deuotion, and a chriſtianlike care towards theſe wicked and ſinfull creatures, are daily inforced to take in a number of theſe diſeaſed people, that otherwiſe would infect many good and honeſt perſons: ſeeking with like care to reſtraine this greeuous infection, and yet the number ſtill increaſeth. It happened very ſeldom in the Hoſpitall of Saint Bartholomewes, whileſt I ſtaied there: amongſt euery twentie ſo diſeaſed, that were taken into the ſaid houſe, which was moſt commonly vpon the Monday, ten of them were infected with Lues Venerea: and therefore how carefully it ought to be looked vnto, let euery man iudge that hath care of his own health, and here I proteſt, that the very cauſe that moued me to ſet forth this booke, is not of vaine glory, neither to incourage ſuch kinde of people to wallow or continue in their beaſtly life, thinking by this booke, or any other whatſoeuer, to be able to deliuer themſelues from this odious ſicknes. But euen in the loue of my countreymen, partly to admoniſh them to amend their liues, and partly to helpe thoſe good people that be infected by eating or drinking, or keeping cōpany vnawares with thoſe diſeaſed perſons: which either for ſhame, dare not bewray it, or for lacke of good Surgeons know not how to remedy it, or for lacke of abilitie, are not able otherwiſe to prouide for the cure of it. And laſt of all to ſhew the way of helpe to cure all ſuch as be infected, and by that meanes, if it may ſo ſtand with the good pleaſure of Almightie God, to ſtop the further ſpreading of the ſame.

And thus I haue by long digreſſion (although not any thing beſides the matter) ſlipped from ſpeaking of the original of this diſeaſe, vnto the complaint of the mightie increaſe thereof, growne in this land, al which I refer vnto the good conſideration of euery diſcreet Reader.

The maner of taking this ſickneſſe, with the cauſes and ſignes thereof. Cap. 2.

How this ſicknes is taken.

This ſickneſſe is ſaid firſt to be ingendred by the vnlawful copulation and accompanying with vncleane women, or common harlots, which although it be for the moſt part true, yet it is not alwaies ſo, nor in all perſons: for I my ſelfe haue knowne, both men and women, greeuouſly infected with this ſicknes, which haue had thoſe parts that bring the moſt ſuſpition thereof, and are moſt ſpeedily infected, free and cleere from all kinde of maladie, or ſhew

of

of any such disease: whereas, if the infection had hapned by that means, those parts should in reasonable likelihood haue béen first touched, as being most apt to putrifie, by reason of the humiditie & loosenes of the part, which engendreth vlcerations of all sorts, apostumes, dolors, putrifactions, and venemous pustules, &c.

I haue also knowne diuers persons infected, who haue had in all other parts of the bodie manifest signes thereof, as dolors, tumors, vlcers, and venemous pustules, &c. And yet in the parts aforesaid, no paine, or any signe thereof: so that their opinion is not to be obserued, which affirme, that this disease is ingendred onely, by the company of vncleane persons: for I haue knowne not many yéeres past, thrée good and honest Midwiues infected with this disease, called Lues Venerea, by bringing abed thrée infected women, of thrée infected children, which infection was chiefly fixed vpon the Midwiues fingers and hands, &c. What should I speake of yong sucking children, whereof diuers haue béen gréeuously vexed with this disease, and some of them a moneth, two, thrée or fower moneths old, and some of them a yéere old, some fower or fiue yéeres old, and some of them sixe or seauen yéeres old, amongst which sort, I thought it good here to note a certaine wench, the daughter of one Sare, of twelue yéeres of age, the which I cured, in the yéere of our Lord 1567. who was greatly infected with this sicknesse in many parts of hir body, hauing thereon painfull nodes or hard swellings and vlcers, with corruption of the bones, and yet no signe in the most suspected parts, neither by reason of debilitie was able to haue committed any such act, but it is not to be doubted, but that she receiued the infection, either from the parents, the which cure of some is supposed vncertaine, whether children begotten by infected parents, may be cured or not: or else she was infected, as diuers are, by sucking the corrupt milke of some infected nurse, of whom I haue cured many, for such milke is ingendred of infected blood, and I may not here in conscience ouerpasse, to forewarne thée good Reader, of such lewde and filthie nurses: for that in the yéere 1583. it chanced that thrée yong children, all borne in this citie of London, all of one parish, or very néere togither, and being of honest parentage, were put to nurse, the one in the countrie, and the other two were nursed in this citie of London: but within lesse than halfe a yéere, they were all thrée brought home to their parents and freends, gréeuously infected with this great and odious disease, by their wicked and filthy nurses: Then their parents séeing them thus miserably spoiled and consumed with extreme paines, and great breaking out vpon their bodies, and being so yong, sicke and weake, vnpossible to be weaned, were forced, as nature doth binde, to séeke by all meanes

Notæ.

A wench being xij. yeeres of age, infected with this sicknes, &c.

Note.

Beware of such nurses.

meanes possible to preserue these poore seely infants, which else had died most pitifully. To be breefe, ere euer those children could be cured, they had infected fiue sundry good & honest nurses: I cured one of the children, and the nurse which gaue it sucke, the other two children & their nurses were also cured by others, but one of the children liued not long after, as I was giuen to vnderstand. Also freendly Reader, I read of late in a certain history, written by *Ambrose Pare*, in his 2. booke, intreating of the causes of Lues Venerea, which history indeed is worthy the rehearsall:

An history of Ambrose Pare.

„ An honest Citizen saith he, granted his most chaste wife, that she should „ nurse the childe which she was lately deliuered of, if she would keepe a „ nurse to be partaker of the trauell and paines: the nurse that she tooke „ by chance, was infected with Lues Venerea, therefore she did presently „ infect the foster childe, and he the mother, and she the husband and he „ two children which he had daily at his table & bed, not knowing of that „ poison which he did nourish in his own body and intrals. But when the „ mother considered and perceiued, that hir childe did not prosper or profit „ by the nourishment, but continually cried and waxed waiward, desired „ me to tell hir the cause of that disease, neither was it any hard matter to „ do, for his body was full of the small pocks, whelks, and venereous „ pustules: and the breasts of the nurses and mother being looked on, were „ eroded with virulent vlcers: and the body of the father and his two „ sonnes, the one about three yeeres, and the other fower yeeres of age, „ were infected with the like pustules and swellings that the childe had: „ therfore I shewed them that they were all infected with Lues Venerea, „ whose beginnings, and as it were prouocations, were spred abroad by „ the nurse that was hired, by hir maligne infection. I cured them all, „ and by the helpe of God, brought them to health, except the sucking „ childe, which died in the cure: and the nurse being called before the ma- „ iestrates, was punished in prison, & whipped closely, and had been pub- „ likely whipped through all the streets of the citie, if it had not been for „ the honor of that vnfortunate family. Thus we see children infected by filthy nurses, and somtimes nurses be infected by giuing sucke to such infected children. And now to returne to my former purpose, the disease, as saith *Nicholas Masa*, whose counsell and direction in the cure of this disease I haue greatly obserued. The disease bicause it hath a flowing matter, being once entred into any part of the body, proceedeth on from part to part, neuer resting vntill it hath corrupted the liuer, with the ill disposition of this infection especially. When it toucheth any such part, as hath in it an apt disposition to admit such infection, as when the acti- on or force of the agent is wrought and imprinted in the patient, fitly affected to receiue the same forme, and so it disperseth it selfe through

the

the whole bodie: likewise this sicknesse is many times bred in the mouth, by eating and drinking with infected persons, and sometimes onely by breathings: and *Almanor* a learned Physition setteth downe for a truth, that this disease may be taken by kissing, and somtimes by lying in the bed with them, or by lying in the sheets after them: also it is said to come by sitting on the same stoole of easement, where some infected person frequenteth, and sometimes such as haue beene cured of this disease, fall into it againe by wearing their olde infected apparell: all which causes of this disease I rather set downe, for that I woulde thereby admonish as many, as shall read this treatise, to be carefull of themselues in this behalfe, and to shun as much as may be, all such occasions. Now all these outward causes being considered, it remaineth that I speak also of the inward causes of the nourishing of this disease, which (as *Nicolas Massa* saith) is the liuer, whose il disposition is as it were the fountaine, roote and spring thereof: for sith in the liuer is made the separation of all the humors of mans body, as by the good temperature and disposition thereof good humors are bred: euen so by the euill disposition thereof, corrupt humors are ingendred, so that from the liuer doth procéede the matter of nourishment, and the faculties of nourishment to al the body, and it is in respect the maintainer of life: and therfore it is not to be doubted (saith he) but that the corruption of the liuer is the roote of this disease. Inward causes of nourishing this disease.

And if it be obiected, that the disease is taken by externall meanes as aforesaid, by kissing, eating and drinking, clothes infected, milke of nurses, &c. and therefore the liuer is not the cause, and so the definition then can not be true: It is answered, that any outward part being once infected, the disease immediately entreth into the blood, & so créepeth on like a canker from part to part, untill it commeth to the liuer, where being once entred, it corrupteth the fountaine of blood, and from thence sendeth forth the infection by the veines into euery part of the body: and thus this may grow at the first, or after the cure used: for if any one part hath béene left unperfectly cured, it may soone returne againe, and make the disease more dangerous and harder to be cured, than it was at the beginning. But to speake more briefly of this matter, there be generally thrée causes of this sicknes, that is to say.

The Primitiue, the Antecedent, and Coniunct cause, which I gather thus. The Primitiue cause is some bodily touching, either of some infected body, as by shéets, or wearing infected apparell, &c. 1. The Primitiue cause.

The antecedent cause is humors, offending in qualitie or quantitie, or both. 2. The Antecedent cause.

The cause coniunct, are those corrupt humors, or that euill qualitie 3. The Coniunct cause.

 that

that resteth and is setled in the parts affected.

The sicknesse it selfe is of diuers men diuersly defined, but the chiefest writers, I meane those which my selfe read, as *Nicholas Massa, &c.*
Nota. do define it to be an affection of the Liuer: but *Ambrose Pare* noteth in the third chapter of his booke, De Morbo Gallico: that it hath his principall seat and place of grosse and slimie fleame infected, with the maligne qualitie of venereous venome, and the originall beginning being taken by a certaine contagious consequence, to creepe into the humors sooner or slower, according to the disposition of the body of euery one. To returne, I said the opinion of some is, that the antecedent cause is the masse of blood contained in the fower humors, which wasteth the spirits: & the effects therof (as I gather) are these, it corrupteth the blood, and poisoneth the whole humors of the body, and breedeth in the parts thereof pains and aches, virulent and malignant vlcers, nodes, or knobby hardnes, foule scabs, tetters, and ringwormes both in the hands and feete, and callous vlcers about the priuy parts: also that impostume in the grinde called Bubo Venereus, likewise a stinking and virulent gonorrhea, or running of the reines, with great paine and difficultie in making their water: Moreouer, venemous pustules and scabs vpon the forehead, browes, face, and beard, and in other parts of the body, as in the corners of the lips, especially in infants: the haires do fall from the head and beard, paines and aches in the head, shoulder blades, hips, thighes and ioints, which pains afflicting most in the night, and ceasing in the day time, a certaine heauines and painfull aking of the body after sleepe, as though they were broken asunder, sometimes a little feauer, and in some a lingring consumption or wasting of the bodie, there followeth also this contagious sicknes, bunchey nodes, & filthy abscessions or apostumes, with corruption of the bones of the head, called Talpa, and vpon the armes and legs called Tophus or Gommata, especially in old sicknesses, hauing their beginning of grosse and slimy fleame: and oftentimes I haue knowne these bones corrupted and rotten, and the flesh round about it sound, nothing at all touched. Further it is to be noted, that the pustules or moist scabs differ in color and disposition, according to the humor, which most ruleth in them: for sometimes they appeere red, puffed vp and swelled, and then it is said blood cheefly ruleth: somtimes they be red without swelling, hauing filthy matter, and a certaine drinesse about them, and then choler beareth rule in them: sometimes they be blew and wan, with grosse matter, and then they proceede most of melancholy: finally, they are somtimes white, broad, and soft, and then fleame hath the dominion. And thus I haue breefly noted what I haue read and found out by experience, concerning the beginning,

spreading,

spreading, causes and signes of this sicknesse, the which I confesse, I should haue more orderly set downe in particular Chapters, with the prognostications, which in some sort are partly omitted. But for that I followed this course of writing in my former bookes, I meane not heere now to alter or change my order and method, which I haue already published: neuerthelesse, I trust no well meaning man shall iustly finde fault with the truth of the matter and maner of curing, &c. Wherefore I will begin first with preparing and purging of the body, &c. Nota.

The way to cure Lues Venerea, beginning first with euacuation. Cap. 3.

THe maner of cure (so far foorth as I meane in this short Treatise to deale with) consisteth of these parts, that is, of euacuation, diet, and vse of vnctions: euacuation is the first of these three to be vsed, namely purgings, letting of blood, and sweating, according to mine owne way & order of curing. Purging first is very necessary, for that many vse to cure this disease onely by euacuation and purging, especially when the sicknesse is newly taken, & the nature of the patient strong and lusty, but we daily finde, that purgings are very seldome sufficient, if the disease haue continued any time, or taken deepe roote, or if there be in the patient any debilitie or weaknes of nature, or much abundance of infected humors or matter, dispersed ouer the whole body.

So according to my former sayings, we vse to begin our cure with preparing and purging of the body, wherein the learned Physition ought to be counselled with: for I read that *Hippocrates*, whose iudgement heerein is vnreprouable, saith: That it is very expedient to purge the digested humor, and in no wise to moue the vnconcocted and raw matter: therefore that which is thicke is to be thinned, and that which is clammie must be absterged, and the obstructed passages are to be opened by conuenient syrups and waters, such like as here presently shall be noted, and the humors being thus ripened, are afterwards to be purged by pils, potions, and other good purgations, according vnto the discretion of the learned: Otherwise it is not meete that euery one should follow his owne aduise and counsell herein. Now presently I thinke good to set downe what preparatiues, pils, and other purgations may conueniently be vsed in this cure, which I haue by long experience and diligent practise obserued and approued, &c.

Preparatiues.

Gualter Bruell.

℞. Syr. Fumar. ℥.iii.
Lupulorum }
Oxymel. simpl. } ana. ℥.j.
Aquæ fumar. }
Lapathi acuti } ana. ℥.iiij.
Lupulorum }
Misce.

Another,

Arceus.

℞. Syr. Fumar. }
Mel. ros. } ana. ℥.j.
Aquæ Fumar. ℥.iij.
Misce.

Another,

Vigo.

℞. Syr. Fumar. minoris ℥.j.
Succ. Endiu. ʒ.vj.
Aquæ Fumar. }
Capil. Vener. } ana. ℥.j.
Misce.

Another,

Clowes.

℞. Syr. Fumar. }
Acetosæ }
Buglos. } ana. ℥.ß.
Capil. Vener. }
Aquæ fumar. }
Scabiosæ } ana. ℥.j.ß.
Misce.

Purgations.

Gualter Bruell.

℞. Diacathol. }
Confect. Hamech. } ana. ʒ.iij.
Sp. Diacarthami ʒ.j.ß.

Elect.

Eeƈt.de ſucco roſ.ʒ.j.
Syr.fumar.℥.j.
Aquæ Lupulorum ℥.iij.
Miſce.

Another.

℞. Caſſiæ fiſtulæ ℥.ß. Vigo.
Diacathol ℥.j.
Eleƈt.de ſucco roſ. ʒ.ij.
Or in the ſtead thereof Confec.hamech.ʒ.ii. make hereof a ſmall potion with the common decoction, &c.

Another,

℞. Senæ orient.℥.i. Clowes.
Paſſularum mund. ℥.ii.
Cinnamo ʒ.iii.
Coriand. } ana.℥.ß.
Galang. }
Polypodii quer. contuſi.℥.ii.
Glycyrrizæ raſæ aniſi ana.℥.ß.
Boile theſe in a quart of running water till the third part be conſumed, then take of this decoction ℥.iii. whereto yee ſhall adde Confeƈt. hamech.ʒ.iii. Diacathol. Eleƈt.In.ma.ana.ʒ.ii. Syr.fumar.℥.j. Miſce.

Other waies of purging by Pils, &c.

Pil.Hermodaƈt.Cochiæ.Aureæ.Fumar.de Aga.de Colocynthi.Rhabarb. the doſes of any of theſe Pils to be taken is ʒ.i. at a time, &c. Ordinary Pils to purge this ſickneſſe.

Pils,

℞. Labdani puri } ana.℥.i. Rondeletius.
Hypociſthidis }
Aloes }
Ambræ } ana.℈.i.
Moſchi }
Argenti viui loti in vino ℥.ii.
Incorporentur ſimul cum Syr.roſ. laxatius & fiant pil. whereof the patient ſhall take euery morning one ſcruple. But theſe Pils muſt not

not be taken before the body be otherwise euacuated, neither any thing else in those daies to be used.

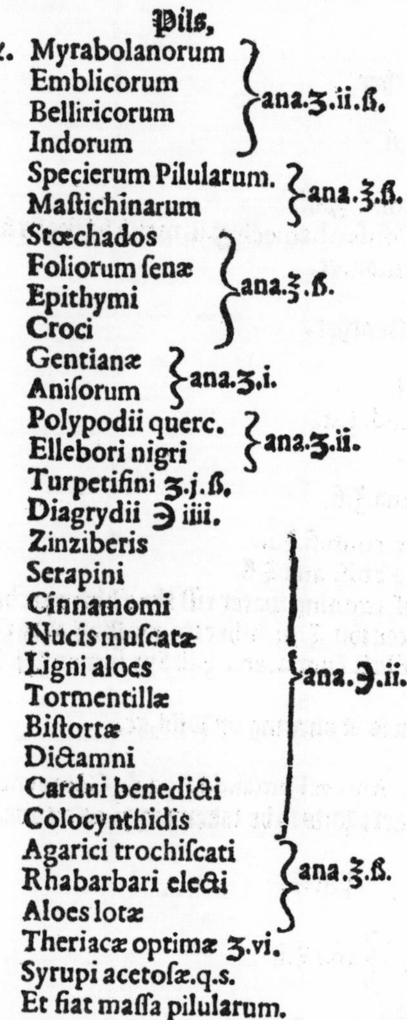

Pils,

Vigo. R. Myrabolanorum
Emblicorum
Belliricorum
Indorum } ana.ʒ.ii.ß.
Specierum Pilularum.
Mastichinarum } ana.℥.ß.
Stœchados
Foliorum senæ
Epithymi
Croci } ana.℥.ß.
Gentianæ
Anisorum } ana.ʒ.i.
Polypodii querc.
Ellebori nigri } ana.ʒ.ii.
Turpetifini ʒ.j.ß.
Diagrydii ℈ iiii.
Zinziberis
Serapini
Cinnamomi
Nucis muscatæ
Ligni aloes
Tormentillæ
Bistortæ
Dictamni
Cardui benedicti
Colocynthidis } ana.℈.ii.
Agarici trochiscati
Rhabarbari electi
Aloes lotæ } ana.℥.ß.
Theriacæ optimæ ʒ.vi.
Syrupi acetosæ.q.s.
Et fiat massa pilularum.

Let the doses be taken at one time ʒ. i. whereof make fiue pils and after them fiue other, &c. And this is the whole some and effect of the preparing and purging of this sicknes as aforesaid. And so héere I will conclude this part, and now I meane to speak of the second kind of euacuation, &c,

A very ſhort note of the maner and order of blood letting in this ſickneſſe. Cap. 4.

CONcerning letting of blood, which is the ſecond kind of euacuation: I hope it may be lawfull for me in ſome ſort to ſpeak, according to mine owne experience and obſeruations héerein.

It is commonly called the opening of a veine, wherein are many obſeruations to be noted, eſpecially theſe thrée: the ſtrength of the body, the conſtitution of aire, and the motion and place of the planets. The ſtrength of the patient is to be conſidered by view of al the actions of the body, that is to ſay, of the Animal actions, of the Vitall actions, & Naturall actions: For if the patient haue his féeling and mouing powers, which is reaſon, imagination, and memory ſound and good, then (as I read) he is ſtrong in his Animal actions.

And likewiſe are his Vitall actions good, if his pulſe be ſtrong, and his reſpiration good, frée, and eaſie. The Naturall actions are concoctions, diſtribution, & aſſimilation: farther I noted of late out of certain learned writers, that the ſignes and tokens are truly taken of the vrine, ſweate, and the excrements of the belly, all which do betoken ſtrength, if they be moſt like to the whole and ſound perſons: and contrariwiſe they argue weakneſſe if they vary, or be very vnlike the ſound and perfect parts. It is moreouer conuenient to looke, that the patient that muſt bléed be neither too yoong nor too old, for children are not commonly let blood before the age of fourtéene yéeres, nor old folkes after thréeſcore, except ſome great cauſe enforce, and then neither age, nor yet the ſigne is much to be regarded. Againe yée ſhall note, that it is not méete to let blood in this ſickneſſe at all times, eſpecially thoſe perſons which are oppreſſed with many cold and raw humors, for ſo by blood letting the humors are made the more crude and rawe, and then the patient thus infected, will be the worſe and harder to be cured. Theſe cauſes I ſay being well conſidered of, with the age and ſtrength of the patient, then it is requiſite that the conſtitution of the aire be alſo obſerued, and the time of the yéere, therefore the aire may not be too hot nor too cold, bicauſe heate diſſolueth and weakneth the ſtrength, and cold congealeth & thickeneth the blood, and hindereth the expulſion of things noiſome: the aire therefore muſt be temperate. And laſtly, touching the motion and place of the planets, it is ſaid to be very dangerous to touch any part of mans body with launce or knife, when the moone hath motion in that ſigne, which

gouerneth

gouerneth the part that should be striken or incised, as to open a veine in the head when the moone is in Aries: or in the necke when it is in Taurus, in the armes the moone being in Gemini, &c. But specially note these thrée rules, if the moone be in Leo, by the which the hart is gouerned, it hath béene thought of many then very dangerous to be let blood at all: if the moone be in Gemini which doth respect the armes then must no veine be touched on the right arme, or on the left.

1. The first veine. Thirdly, thrée veines are most usually to be opened: the first is called Cephalica, that is the head veine, which is the vpper veine that appéereth in the bowing of the arme, and that for the paines and diseases of the head.

2. The second veine. The second is called Hepatica, or the liuer veine, which also appéereth at the bowing of the arme, and serueth for the obstructions, and other affects of the liuer.

3 The third veine. The third is called Mediana, that is, the middle veine, which is made of both those aforesaid, and respecteth both head and liuer, and is opened with lesse danger. To the former rules (which note as the fourth) that on the day of the change or full moone, or on the next day following, or going before, letting of blood is not good, except (as I said before) that there be some other vehement necessitie, and great perill doth require, then we may not in any wise tarrie, or stay till the signe be good: but presently open the veine, least peraduenture the patient, which should be let blood, do happen to die in the meane space. For truly I haue séene and knowen many restored to their perfect health, by letting of blood, when the signe hath béene accounted and knowen to be very dangerous and ill: and likewise I haue séene others that were so curious, that they would in no wise let blood, when the signe was in the place, but after they did repent themselues, when it was too late. Thus you haue héere briefly the two first kinds of euacuation. The third which is sweating, shall be handled héereafter, when I shew the vse of vnctions. Now presently followeth that I also speake somwhat as concerning diet, &c.

The order of diet in this cure. Cap. 5.

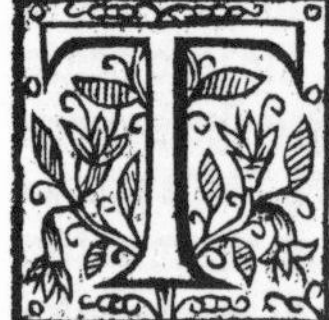

Diet to be vsed. This third part, which I purpose héere to speake of in the cure of this sicknes, is diet. Wherein first it is to be obserued, that the meates which the patient must vse, ought to be of easie digestion, and of good nourishment, and such as ingender fewest superfluities and excrements, as white bread not too much leauened, not too stale, nor too new, except there be some other speciall intention and purpose:

pose: the flesh must neither be very yong nor very old, nor too moist as porke or lambe, nor too dry, as béefe and venison. These following are very good, weathers mutton, veale, lambe, and kid, being fed in drie grounds, yong hares and rabbets, chickens, capons, hens, partriges, feasants, and birds of the woods and mountains: any of these may be giuen to the sicke patient, either rosted or sodden, without salt or spice, except some speciall cause require the contrarie. But yet you may boile in your broths prunes, raisons of the sun, and currants, with spinage, parsley, and white béetes: and your broths must be also thickened with white bread, and seasoned with veriuice, &c. Swines flesh, salt meates, géese and ducks, and such wilde foules as liue in waters, are not wholsome in this case, but rather do great hurt: fish is not greatly to be liked of, bicause it is cold and moist, neither chéese, for it is hard of digestion: egs potched, or put in broths, are very good: all rawe waterish and cold fruits are to be eschewed, for they ingender rawe humors and putrifactions: and swéete wines in this case, saith *Nicholas Massa*, are not to be vsed: for they cause obstructions, and also make great heate and boiling in the bodie, and old wine doth not nourish: but generally I haue found good small and stale ale in the cure of this sicknes best. And ye shall specially obserue in this way of curing, that if the patient be weake of body, that then euery morning before ye enter him into the vnction, and so to sweat in his bed, that you giue vnto him some good caudell or aleberrie, as this or the like, ℞. Ale, sugar, the yelke of an egge or two, and the crust of white bread, boile all these togither, and so drinke it hot: or else in the stead of a caudell or aleberry, you may giue them to drinke the broth of a chicken or mutton, or else a messe of new milke sod with some sugar: this doth greatly comfort and strengthen the sicke patient, and prouoketh sweat the sooner: and note that such as be great eaters and drinkers, and immoderate vsers of women: and otherwise be disordered persons are vnfit for this cure, and their healths almost are not to be looked for. But when any man shall enter into this diet and cure, there must be chosen a fit place for the patient to lie in, frée from corrupt aires, such (I mean) as be in moist marish grounds, stinking ditches and lakes, laystals, riuers and springs, &c. And let your chamber be close, and voide of open aire, and well rectified with swéete sauours and smels. And thus much as touching the third part of this cure, which respecteth dieting of the patient. And now followeth the vse of vnctions or ointments, and that is as it were, the perfection of the whole cure, &c.

The maner and order of annointing, with other necessarie obseruations to be considered of in this cure. Cap. 6.

THe fourth part of the cure of this disease, so far forth (as I haue said) I haue purposed to deale with, consisteth chiefly in vnctions, which part I meane héere through Gods assistance, truly and plainly to set downe, and first of all I thinke it best to expresse the way and order of annointing with the vnctions made of quicksiluer, which is thus. The chamber being first prouided in a decent place, as is said in the Chapter going before, then let the patient be prepared to bed, and if it be in the sommer time, then let the chamber be strowed with rushes, the leaues of willowes, violets, roses, baies, vine leaues, and other coole and swéete herbes, sometimes being sprinkled with vineger and rose water. But in the winter time, and in very colde weather, let there be made a good fire of coles, rather in a pan, than in a chimney. Now héere fréendly Reader, I haue thought it good vpon speciall occasion, to note vnto you the great and perilous dangers which my selfe haue séene and knowen to follow vpon a sudden, by reason of the venemous cloudy vapors of charcoles, which hath smothered and strangled diuers and sundry persons, being placed in close chambers, before the coles were first throughly burned in the open aire, or in a chimney: and then after they be well burned, they may be safely vsed without all danger: and hauing a pan of coles thus prepared, then before you annoint him or hir whatsoeuer they be, giue them to drinke some good caudle, which will comfort and strengthen the stomacke, as is before said, and procure sweate the sooner: then next let him be annointed against a good fire of coles, and then they must rub or chafe it in well with their owne hands, if it be possible their strength will serue, & those parts or places that are to be annointed, are first the soles of the féete, and so vp to the knees, also the thighes, buttocks, loines, and share bones, and likewise annoint both the armes, and vnder the arme holes, and the shoulder blades: but in any wise, as néere as you can, touch not the head, neither come néere any other principall parts with the vnction, as the belly, for thereby truly I haue séene gréeuous accidents to follow, and oftentimes death, as hereafter shall be declared. The annointing being thus finished, let a warme shéete be put round about the patient, and a double kercher well warmed, and bound about his head, and so

Nota.

so couer him in his bed, with as many clothes as he is well able to beare: but if therewith he cannot sweate orderly, as you would desire, then applie to the soles of his féete, legs, thighes, and to both his sides, very hot bricks well wrapped in warme double clothes, or else bottels filled with very hot water, or in stéede thereof wodden bores, of twelue inches long, and made round, with a lid at one end, and hollow like a pipe, and well plated in the inside, wherein you shall put a long round péece of hot iron, so big as will easily go into the bore, and then put on the lid, and wrap thrée or fower of these bores in hot clothes, and applie them to the places aforenamed: and when the patient doth begin to sweat, that then you shall haue in a readinesse, a clocke watch, or houre glasse, that you be not deceiued of the time in their sweating, and then halfe an houre before they haue sweat out the full time, be it either two or thrée houres or more, as the necessitie of the cause requireth, then begin to abate his clothes by little and little, and so let him or hir coole by degrées, but take héede of sudden or ouer hastie cooling: moreouer, if it so fall out in the time of his sweating, that he be greatly desirous to drink, then you may admit him ale warmed with a toste, or else warme posset ale, being put into a glasse which hath a long pipe, and let it be giuen him by his kéeper, for himselfe may not put his hands out of the bed, to giue himselfe drink, for feare of colde: also if he chance to grow faint in his sweating, you may safely giue him now and then of Manus Christi, and likewise let him smell to rose water & viniger, and cast it suddenly into his face: and when his sweats be orderly finished and done, and his shirt that he sweate in is well dried and warmed, then let him put it on quickly, and also a waste cote, or warme dublet, and about his necke a halfe shéete warmed, and kéepe his head likewise very warme, and let him sit vp in his bed, then giue him some warme broths, &c. He must be thus annointed and ordered, two or thrée daies togither or more, as you sée occasion, vntill the fluxe of flegmatike matter doth begin to flow from the mouth moderately, which doth happen commonly within two, thrée, or fower daies, &c. Then cease from annointing, for otherwise it is very dangerous, as shall be declared. This being thus done, then will the gums, chéekes, toong and throteranckle, vlcerate and swell, which may safely be cured, by this maner and order following. First, let there be bounde vnder his chin, a double linnen cloth, and pinned vp to his kercher, and then wash and gargarise his mouth with new milke, wherein you may séeth a few violet leaues, and columbine leaues, and syrup of violets, and sometime this following,

A good meanes to cause sweate.

Beware of colde, and of an euill keeper, the one is a deadly enimie, and the other is a pestilent euill in this sicknesse.

Gargarismes to coole the mouth in the beginning.

℞. Aquæ hord. } ana.q.s.
Mel.ros. }

Syr. violacei q.s.

Or else take,

Aquæ periclymen. ℥.vi.
Diamoron. ℥.j.
Mel.rof. ℥.ij.
Misce.

Use these two or thrée daies, and then let the mouth, gums and throte be throughly mundified and clensed with this lotion, which I haue proued to be singular good, &c.

A very good lotion. Clowes.

℞. Aquę fontanæ lib.xii.
Vini albi lib.iiij.
Mellis com. lib.ij.
Aluminis rochæ lib.ß.
Hordei contusi m. ii.
Sumach ℥.j.
Corticis granatorum ℥.iiij.
Saluiæ
Fœniculi
Rubii
Periclym.
Equiseti
Rorismarini } ana. m.ij.
Foliorum plantaginis
Polygoni
Summitatum Rubi.
Quinque folii
Fragar.
Aquilegiæ } ana.m.j.
Cochleariæ m.ij.

Boile all these togither, till one part be consumed, then take it from the fire and straine it, and so kéepe it to your vse. The mouth must be washed, and the throte gargarised with this lotion thrée or fower times a day, vntill the paines be ceased, the téeth fastened, and the vlcers of the mouth and throte clensed and healed. But if the vlceration in the mouth and throte be so rebellious, that it will not yéeld to these remedies, as oftentimes I haue séene: then I vse to touch the vlcers of the mouth, two or thrée times, or more, with Aqua fallopii, or some other good Mercury water, or else with Vnguentum Ægyptiacum being first warmed, & afterward you may safely cure it with my foresaid lotion, wherunto now and

and then I do ad Mel rosa.q.s. & then after the vlcers in the mouth be wel mundified & clensed, I do after vsually cure the same with my lotion only. I know I might here set down a number of other lotions tending to the same purpose, but I will omit them. And thus briefly haue I spoken of the maner of annointing, & the order of sweating, and the cure of the mouth: which with great foresight, care, & diligence is to be looked vnto: for otherwise if it be neglected, then doth follow most commonly great & dangerous accidents, & this may come either by the disobedience & vnrulines of the patient, or else through the ignorance or negligence of the Surgeon, not regarding the malice and sharpnesse of the flure, whereby it doth happen often times, that some haue béene eaten cleane through the chéeks, & also haue had their Vuula therby taken away, by the means héereof they haue lost their spéeches and voices, others haue lost their téeth and mandible or iaw withall, insomuch they were neuer able afterward to receiue any food to sustaine them, but onely with a spoone vntill their dying day. Therefore I am héere to aduertise thée good Reader, to be very wary of such carelesse and ignorant Surgeons, for those dangers and causes before spoken of: likewise I do againe admonish all good and skilfull Artists, to eschew and beware as much as possible they may, all such disobedient, vnruly, disordered, and vnfortunat patients, which are oftentimes the onely cause of their owne misery, and so shame and discredit vnto their Physition or Surgeon: wherfore at the beginning of such great and immoderat fluxes at the mouth, defer no time, but with all spéed aske counsell of the learned Physition or Chirurgeon, and be nothing ashamed so to do, least as (I haue said) you repent when it is too late, and excuse your selfe, with noddies had I wist: but where no conference can presently be had, there prepare thy selfe to make this clyster héere following,

Nota.

The disease is alwaies to be accounted vncurable, where the patient is disobedient and will not be gouerned by his Physition or Surgeon.

℞. Maluæ
Parietariæ } ana.m.i.
Mercurialis
Rad. althææ. m. ß.

Boile these with a weathers head being first well chopped, and then put into a sufficient quantity of water vntill the flesh be tender, and that the bones be ready to separate from the flesh, and take of this decoction lib.i. then adde to it,

Oleor. rosa.
Chamæmelini } ana. ℥. ß.
Diacatholici ℥. ß.
Diaphœnici ℥. vi.

Luteorum

The clister. Luteorum ouorum num. ii.

Misce & fiant clyster.

And if it so chance that a clister cannot be presently made, then with spéed administer a suppository or two, which you may make thus,

R. Mellis com. }
Pulueris hieræ } ana.q.s.

Or els take

Mellis com. }
Salis com. } ana.q.s.
Misce.

Boile any of these till it be thicke and hard, and then make it round, greater at the one end than at the other, and in length thrée, fower, or fiue inches, and when you administer it, annoint the fundament with Ol.amygdalorum, or with Ol. rof. or Butyri recentis q.s. and also let him drinke of a caudell, wherein you may in such extremities put the powders of

Nucis muscatæ }
Maceris }
Cinnamomi }
Garyophyllorum }
Coral.rub. } ana.q.s.
Bol.orient. }
Fol.rof.rub. }
Corticis granator. }
Florum balaustior. }

And also giue them to drinke of Almond milke, and of a Cinnamon water, and for to strengthen and warme his stomack, giue hir or him at times, conserue of Roses ℥.ii. Mithridat. ℥.j. Misce. And morouer, to helpe to preuent these euill accidents of the mouth, let the patient hold in his mouth Butyri recentis, and also now and then in like maner Ol. amygdalorum dul.q.s. they do helpe to mollifie the hard swelling of the chéekes, & will be a means greatly to preserue the mouth from the malice and sharpnesse of those vile and vicious humors, which corrode and eate the parts: these likewise are profitable helpes to repell and draw backe great fluxes at the mouth: first let there be set certaine cupping glasses vpon the shoulders, and vpon the muskles of Hypochondria, or vpon the loines, and vpon both the buttocks: and it is very good also to vse somtimes frictions or rubbings, and likewise in great extremities I haue séene profit by the vse of Vesicatories to blister the shoulders and hinder parts, which Vesicatories are made thus,

R. Cau-

℞. Cantharidum
Euphorbii
Sinapis } ana.℥.ß.
Mellis ℥.i.

Vesicatories to blister.

Aceti & fermenti, quod satis sit, accipiantur & fiat vesicatorium.

Or this,

℞. Cantharidum
Aceti & fermenti } ana.q.s.

All these are necessary helps being vsed in due time.

Heere also note, that often times it chanceth the patient hath little flux at the mouth, but onely it floweth altogither downward by stoole, and that abundantly, and this may chance either by disorder of the patient in taking of cold, or else by applying of the vnction vpon the belly, which fluxe in some hath easily beene staied, and the patient so perfectly cured, and neuer had any fluxe at the mouth: but in some it hath beene staied with great difficultie and much danger. Againe in other some it could neuer be staid, but they haue died with the extremity of the flux. And heere yee shall obserue & note, that I haue applied the vnction being very strong and good vnto sundry bodies, ten and twelue times togither, and yet by no maner of meanes I could bring them to any fluxe, either at the mouth or downewards: but in such fluxes aforesaid giue the patient also to drinke of Cow milke, and of Gotes milke, wherin hath been oftentimes quenched hot gads of steele, adding thereto also a peece of fine sugar, and a cup or two of Ipocras may be permitted, as by experience I haue often seene.

Nota.

And it is good to take Conseruę prunellorum, conf. ros. antiq. ana.℥.j. and in great necessity we haue vsed to giue the patient Aqua composita, or of Master *Kebles* water published in the end of this booke, applying continually to the bottome of his belly, hot trenchers well wrapped in warme double clothes, and also put a double hot cloth to his fundament, hauing prepared in readines a close stoole, vnder the which yee shall set a pan or pot with hot water, wherein shall be boiled these herbes following,

℞. Fol. lauri
Absinthii
Maioranæ
Menthæ
Saluiæ
Chamæmeli } ana.m.i.

A bath of herbs good in immoderate fluxes of the belly by reason of the anointings.

Anethi

Anethi
Meliloti
Thimi
Fœniculi
Rorismarini } ana.m.i.
Hyssopi
Origani
Fol.ros.rub.

Boile these in a sufficient quantity of water, & whilest he sitteth at the stoole, let his bed be new made and warmed with a warming pan, and take heed of cold in any wise, &c. And thus briefly I cōclude this part. Next I will set downe the best approoued vnctions, that my selfe haue knowen in all the time of my practise for many yeeres, with other remedies, which I haue also found to be very profitable helpes for the cure of this sicknesse, and then with as much breuity as I can, I will conclude this order of cure, &c.

Of the nature and properties of Quicksiluer, with the excellent vertues of the same.

Cap. 7.

I Haue thought it most meete and conuenient, for the better vnderstanding of all yong students in Chirurgerie, briefly to set downe the nature and propertie of Quicksiluer, with the singular vertues of the same, &c. *Nicholas Massa* in his booke de Morbo Gallico affirmeth, that quicksiluer is hot and moist, and that the nature of quicksiluer is to penetrate, dissolue, and prouoke sweate and fluxes at the mouth and fundament, &c. Of the contrarie opinion is *Auicen*, saying that it is cold in the second degree: and to proue his opinion to be good, he citeth an historie of an Ape, which did drinke quicksiluer, and so died, by reason thereof the body was dissected, and there was found besides the hart, a great quantitie of congealed blood, which did arise (say they) of no other cause, but onely of the coldnes of the quicksiluer. But *Marianus Sanctus Barolitanus* saith, he saw a woman, which for certaine griefes and diseases, tooke halfe a pound of quicksiluer at many times, which she auoided at hir belly without any hurt. *Ambrose Pare* noteth very well an history of an Apothecarie, which to stay the thirst of his feuer, tooke a vessell full of quicksiluer, thinking it had been water, and within a few howers died, he auoiding

An history.

great

great quantitie of the quicksiluer by the fundament: and after that he was opened, there was found in his stomacke a pound: and besides this there was likewise found congealed blood: and this is by some obiected and alleged onely to prooue the coldnes of quicksiluer. But these arguments and reasons I thought to be very weake and of no force. For *Antonius Musa* approoueth it good, and to be a most singular and safe remedie to be giuen to yong children, hauing tender and delicate bodies, for the cure of wormes in their bodies, being a most dangerous and deadly maladie. *Almanor* a learned doctor of physicke saith, that quicksiluer is hot, and by his heate doth warme and make thin the humors being well prepared, and doth expell them by the uppermost and outwarde parts of the body. *Paulus* also doth affirme it to be hot and moist in the fourth degree, to whose opinion the said *Almanor* agreeth, and is wholy against *Auicen*, who maketh it cold in the second degree. Also a note deliuered unto me by a friend, of the nature and qualitie of quicksiluer, according to the minde of *Paracelsus*, in his booke called Congere, where he writeth De transmutatione Metallorum, saith he: "They that iudge quicksiluer to be cold and moist of nature are deceiued, and conuinced by their owne error, for naturally it is hot and moist: for that maketh it to continue in his flowing and liquidnes: for if it were cold and moist, it would alwaies haue forme of congealed water, as ice, and would be hard and solid: besides that it would require fire to melt it as other mettals do, which it doth not, but floweth of his naturall heate, &c. Many men are of many opinions, and allege great reasons to prooue quicksiluer to be cold. But it falleth out, that common experience prooueth the contrarie. For this my selfe doth know most assuredly, that quicksiluer being compounded with Axungia porcina, vnguentum Dialthææ, vulpinum, Aregon, Agrippæ, Genistæ, also Oleum laurinũ, Terebinthinæ, Liliorum, Chamæmelinum, Anethinum, Rosaceum, Lumbricorum, & Hyperici, &c. and such other emolliant and dissoluing remedies. By these meanes I haue resolued nodes and hard swellings, with great comfort unto the parts affected, and so haue cured many, though the griefe were old and of long continuance: and may be performed of any, being (as I haue said) artificially handled, otherwise it is as a sword put into a mad mans hand. But I do truly affirme, that quicksiluer is most profitable for the cure of Lues Venerea, being as it were first mortified & killed with Succus Limonum, succus saluiæ, succus ros. Oleum laurinum, iuniperi, axungia porcina, acetum vini, aqua vitæ, sputum hominis ieiun. oxymel. squiliticum, &c. Thus I say, quicksiluer being sufficiently killed, may then be compounded with the foresaid vnguents and oiles, and other gums and powders, as heerafter in the composition

Nota.

of the vnctions shall be declared. Then shall you finde that the vnctions made with quicksiluer haue great and precious vertues, and it is most true that their opinions ought not to be regarded, which speake so maliciously against the vnctions made with quicksiluer, onely of enuie, to the intent to make this maner of curing séeme odious vnto the world. But for my part, without further obiections to the contrarie, let euery man speake and iudge according as he knoweth and findeth: and this I say most truly, that I yet did neuer sée, but that the profit surmounted the hurt, being diligently and carefully vsed, then I suppose no man was yet euer endamaged thereby, if they speake truly: and so I conclude with the sayings of *Vigo*, that I know no reason why some men should thus condemne medicines made with quicksiluer, séeing that many remedies made with quicksiluer (being so noble a thing as it is) are found in the bookes of ancient and late writers, in the curing of scabs, salt fleam, tetters and ring wormes, &c. But it is said, the cause why they are so headstrong in opinion, or as it were sworne enimies against vnctions made with quicksiluer, truly this is one of their chiefe reasons, to proue their opinion to be good. First they say they be very dangerous & strong, and so cause malignant accidents, and vlcerations in the mouth and gums, toong and throte, with continuall fluxe of flegmatike matter day and night running, whereby happeneth painfull watching, lacke of appetite, with dolour in the iawes, and such other infirmities, which they say is so true, that nothing can be more true. It is answered by the authoritie of *Hippocrates*, that extreme remedies are to be vsed against extreme diseases: for (say they) be there not purgations made very strong, by reason of Eleborus and Scammony, and such like, which hurt the stomacke and other parts, and shall they vtterly be refused, bicause they are noisome? It is supposed not, for by their contraries they are and may be made medicinable: euen the same and the very like proues are there of the vnctions made with quicksiluer. I know full well, it will be obiected against me, as it hath béene against others that were men of great learning and iudgement, that my learning and knowledge héerin, is not to be compared with those men, which hold the contrarie opinion, I grant it to be true, and I would indéede hold their opinions to be good also, but that daily experience hath taught me to the contrarie. And I say with *Guido*, we be children sitting in the necke of a giant, by which meanes we can sée whatsoeuer the giant can sée. And thus haue I obserued and often approued, that the nature and propertie of the vnctions made with quicksiluer, doth prouoke sweate, and emptieth the cause of this disease, somtimes sensible and somtimes insensible, and the blood is thereby purged from infection, and all the parts of the body are

clensed

clensed from superfluous humors, so that good humors in their places are bred, and they do returne againe unto their naturall course and disposition, as we daily find true by experience. But yet beware that too litle of the unction do not deceiue thee in annointing, neither be too bold with the applying of too much of it at a time. Also you must obserue that your frictions or rubbings be done according to the discretion of the skilfull Surgeon and strength of the patient, that is to say moderately, and not too forcibly or ouer roughly, for feare of shutting of the pores, neither too mildly or gently, but in a reasonable meane: for otherwise it will not sufficiently pearse or enter the pores of the skin. Likewise (as I haue before said) beware of the disordered patient, and of the aire, of meates and of drinks: for by such meanes many haue beene defrauded of their healths, and after few daies haue fallen againe into this sicknes, and somtimes ioined with a worse, and more hard to be cured, as the dropsie, &c. There is no certaine time to be limited for the number of the daies, in the applying of the unction, neither how much in quantitie thereof is to be used at a time, but it is necessarie to procede after the strength of the patient, and the force of the unction, and the continuance of the sicknes. These obseruations being skilfully accomplished, and all things aforesaid diligently noted, the mouth and gums healed, and the teeth fastened, then let the patient haue cleane and fresh clothes, as before I haue admonished, and likewise change their sheetes, and not before, except the flux do flow too abundantly. Last of all let them be purged with some conuenient purgation, meete to purge away the relicts remaining of the disease. This done, let the patient be let blood within a day or two, and chose some good sweete aire to remaine in for a space, using a moderate order of diet with conuenient meats and drinks, &c.

A note or obseruation of certaine speciall cures of this disease, called Lues Venerea, by vnctions and other approoued remedies, as followeth. Cap. 8.

FRiendly Reader, I haue thought it not amisse, for the warrantise of this maner of cure, and credit of this booke, to set downe certaine speciall cures performed by me, according to the order of this booke. In the yeere of our Lord 1579. the seuenth of Aprill, was brought unto me, a man of the age of twentie and six yeeres, greeuously ouergrowne with this sicknesse aforenamed, wherewith he had béene infected for the space of fiue yéeres, he had vpon his head a mightie great node, which did corrupt the bones through both the tables, his throte and the rofe of his mouth was déepely infected and eaten with euill vlcers of harde curation, in such sort, that his drinke did come oftentimes out of his nose. He had Tophos and painful hard swellings vpon his legs and armes, so that the two great bones of both his legs, commonly called the shin bones, were with the malice of this sicknesse corrupted and eaten very déepely in certaine places, so that they were for the most part taken away: he had also vpon his brest a very great node, and extreme aches in his ioints, which depriued him of his sléepe, and weakned him very much. This séemed to me so hard a cure, that I would not make them any warrantise or promise of his recouery: but it was the first thing they demanded at my hande, to warrant the cure, and likewise would néedes know of me, by what day I could cure him: vnto whose vnreasonable demands and requests, I answered and said, it was not in me to performe, nor in any other person whatsoeuer: for I sawe that the cure would be troublesome and dangerous vnto the patient, and also great trauell vnto me, and for that his sicknes was great and of continuance, and in a body féeble, and of an ill constitution. Notwithstanding, I promised to do the best I could, so far as reason and experience would lead me: so he was well contented to yéeld himselfe into my hands, and I being not altogither in despaire of his recouerie, for as much as oftentimes we do sée, that beyond all expectation very hard and desperate cures are accomplished and brought to perfect health, &c. But now to speake againe of this cure, which I performed in this order following,

First, hauing prouided for him a conuenient lodging, then I did giue him euery morning for six daies togither, this preparatiue, the which I haue also described before in Cap. 3.

The preparatiue.

℞. Syr. fumar.
Buglos.
Acetosæ
Capil. Vener. } ana. ℥. ß.
Aquæ fumar.
Scabi. } ana. ℥. j. ß.
Misce.

This done, I gaue him the seuenth day, at seauen of the clocke in the morning, this potion following, which did worke wonderfull well, and little offended his stomacke, neither greatly troubled his bodie in the working,

℞. Senæ

The purgation.

℞. Senæ orient. ℥.i.
Seminis anisi
Coriandri
Glycyrrhizæ
Polypod.quer.con.
Galangæ } ana.℥.ß.
Passularum mundat. ℥.ii.
Cinnamomi ʒ. ij.

Boile all these togither in a quart of running water, till the third part be consumed, then take of this decoction ℥.iij. Confect.hamech. ʒ.iij.diacathol.Electuarij Indi ana.ʒ.ij. Syr.fumar.℥.j.Misce. After his bodie was thus prepared and purged, two daies after I toke from him seven ounces of blood from the liver veine of the right arme, that is to say, by reason of his weaknesse, fower ounces in the morning, and three ounces at fower a clocke in the afternoone, which blood looked like unto the colour of glasse, and somwhat thicke and slimy, like unto a mucilage. This also done, I prepared for him to drinke morning and evening, this purging drinke following, ℥. vj. at a time, being warmed, and I so continued it six weekes, only somtimes in the weeke staied a day and somtimes two, without taking any of it, and somtimes he toke it but once a day, as it wrought with him more or lesse. By this drinke and the meanes aforesaid, the malicious humors, which before did continually flow into the parts of the body, and greatly tormented and vexed the patient, were (I say) very much diminished, and that did agree very well with him, and did nothing offend his stomacke, and it furthered greatly the cure, whilest the ulcers were in clensing, and the corrupt bones in scaling. The order of making this decoction is thus,

The liuer veine opened

The decoction or purging drinke.

℞. Ligni sancti lib.j.
Cortic.eiusdem ℥.vi.
Sarsæ parillæ ℥.iiij.
Seminis anisi ℥.j.
Glycyrrhizæ rasæ ℥.i.ß.
Passularum mundat. ℥.iiii.
Senæ orient. ℥.iiii.
Hermodact.
Stœchados } ana.℥.i.
Turpeti opt. ℥. ß.
Polypod.querc. contus. ℥.iii.

Card.

Card. benedic.
Capil. Vener.
Epithymi
Chamæpityos } ana. pu.ii.
Cinnamomi. ℥.i.
Sacchari lib.ß.

Infuse these 24. houres in Aquæ purif. & vini albi. ana. lib.x.

This was boiled vpon an easie fire of coles, till the third part was consumed, and in the cooling was put in of fine Mithridate ℥.ß. and so I strained it: ye shall note that in bodies of a hot constitution, there was left out the Mithridate. I did vse this drinke vntill I had remooued all the corrupt bones, and clensed the foule and filthy vlcers. Onely ye shall further obserue, that when he purged too much, we left off the vse of this drinke, according as I haue before declared, more or lesse as we saw good occasion. All things being orderly performed, then I did apply vnto certaine knots and hard swellings, being laide vpon diuers parts of his bodie, this plaister following,

℞. Emplast. de Meliloto Mesui
Oxycro. } ana. ℥. iiij.
Empl. Vigonis cum Mercurio ℥. vi.
Misce.

And aboue the bones which were corrupted, I did lay round about the sound parts this defensiue,

A defensiue.

℞. Emplast. Diachalciteos lib.ß.
Olei rof. rub.
Myrtillorum } ana. ℥.i.
Succor. plantag.
Solatri } ana. ℥.ß.
Aceti rof. ℥.ß.
Albuminum ouorum num.ii.
Misce.

Hauing applied this defensiue round about the corrupt and hard swelling, then I laid vpon euery node, the white caustick or ruptorie, which I did spread on lint very thicke, and thus with defending, conuenient rowling and bolstering, I bound it thereto, the which caustick continued in working the space of fower or fiue houres: then with all spéede I did hasten the fall of the eschars, with this vnguent,

Vnguentum populeum simpl. to remooue the eschars.

℞. Axungiæ porcinæ lib.ii.
Oculorum populi lib.ß.
Vini albi lib.i.

Let

Let all these rest togither the space of seuen daies, and then boile all togither vntill the wine be consumed, and then straine it, and kæpe it in a cleane vessell: when I had herewith remoued the eschars, and discouered the corrupt and rotten bones: I did then euery day after dresse those græued parts with hot Vnguentum Ægyptiacum, which did not onely helpe greatly to scale the corrupt and rotten bones, but also did subdue and take away the spungeous flesh, which continually did rise in these vncleane vlcers, and it did moreouer correct the malice, and consume filthy humors, which did continually flow to the vlcered parts, and I found much profit in the scaling of the bones with this medicine: but you must defend the fleshy and rawe parts specially in delicate and tender bodies,

℞. Aquæ vitæ or the spirits of wine ℥.vi.
Vitrioli albi crudi ℥.i.
Mellis ros. lib.i.

Boile all these on a gentle fire to the thicknesse of a syrup, and then with pledgets dipped in the same, being vsed very hot vnto the græued parts, once euery day. And for that this patient was in great debilitie, I vsed also euery dressing, afore I applied on the pledgets aforesaid, certain hot steuphs of white wine and Aquæ vitæ, especially on the head, and after these bones were scaled and remoued away, and the vlcers purely clensed, then I administred vnto him this vnction following, which is as it were a most pretious antidote for the curing this disease,

The vnction.

℞. Axungiæ porcinæ lib.j.
Olei lauri ℥.vj.
Argenti viui ℥.v. extincti cum succo saluiæ q.s.
Oleorum Irini, Chamæmeli, Lumbricorum, Ros., Mastich. ana.℥.j.
Theriacæ opt. ℥.ß.
Vnguenti Martiati, Vulpi. ana.℥.ij.
Dialthææ composit., Genistæ ana.℥.j.
Terebinthinæ Venet.℥.j.ß.
Lithargyrij auri ℥.iij.
Cerusæ ℥ j.ß.
Plumbi vsti ℥.j.

Clowes.

Mastichis

Mastiches }
Myrrhæ } ana.℥.ß.
Olibani }
Nucis muscatæ }
Maceris } ana.ʒ.vj.
Caryophyllorum }
Moschi boni ʒ.ß.being dissolued in olei ros.q.s.
Aquæ vitæ ℥.ij.
Misce,& fiat linimentum secundum artem.

With this vnction I annointed him according to the order which before is described, and I finished the rest of the cure with vnguents,plaisters, lotions, gargarismes, and other meete and conuenient remedies in this booke plentifully set down. After I had proceeded thus far in the cure, then I purged him again as before said, & so let him rest frō the vse of all medicines for the space of ten daies, to see if the disease would offer to returne againe, and at the ten daies end I did giue him for the more perfection of his cure, considering the continuance and greatnes of his sicknesse, for the space of one and twenty daies the prescribed drinke, which he did take three times a day,℥.vi. at a time, that is to say,at seauen of the clocke in the morning, and at fower of the clock in the after noone,and lastly at eight of the clock at night: he did drinke at his dinner and supper small ale, his bread was made of the finest wheat being crustie,and sometimes he did eat of bisket bread made of fine flower, kneaded with this decoction, whereunto was added suger q.s. with a few Coriander seedes, and sometimes Aniseeds, and Fenell seeds: his meat was somtimes mutton,capon, hen, chicken,rabbets, &c.Also it is good to eate feasant,partridge,and blacke birds, &c: at the beginning he was allowed two meales a day, but in the end at night he went supperlesse to bed, onely he had giuen him a few raisons of the sunne and almonds blanched, also he did sweat euery weeke one hower or two: and when the one and twenty daies were expired,fower daies after I did open the liuer veine on the left arme, and I did take from him ℥.viii. of blood,and by this order and way of curing he was perfectly healed through the helpe and goodnes of almightie God.

A smith cured of this disease called Robert Clare.

Also some six and twenty yeeres ago I cured on *Robert Clare* a Smith dwelling at town Malling in Kent, he being a man of fifty yeeres old, which was infected with this disease for the space of twelue yeeres, and was a noted man,and commonly known to haue this disease called Lues Venerea, so that no man that knew him would either eat or drinke with him, otherwise I would not haue thus noted him to the world: he had vpon his head, and in diuers places of his face corrosiue, virulent,

and

and malignant vlcers with corruption of the bones, especially on his head and his nose, so that his voice had but a very bad sound, he had other hard swellings and painfull prickings vpon his armes and legs, and also vpon his ioints, which tormented him sore in the night: notwithstanding he had béene a long time in cure with diuers Surgeons, which with this vnction following, and other conuenient remedies appertaining to this cure, which I haue published in this booke, I did perfectly make him whole, and so continued vntill his dying day, which was many yéeres after he was by me perfectly cured and healed,

The vnction.

℞. Axungiæ porcinæ lib.i.
Olei laurini ℥.iiii.
Olei petrolei
Olei lumbricorum } ana.℥.i.
Vnguenti dialthææ
Vnguenti Martiati } ana.℥.ii.
Axungiæ caponis ℥.ii.
Gum. ammoniaci
Opoponacis
Bdellii } ana.℥.i.
Aluminis vsti ℥.ß
Argenti viui ℥.iiii.
Misce, & fiat linimentum secundum artem, &c.

There néedeth no further proofe or authoritie to trie the goodnes of this vnction, and the rest héere by me prescribed, than experience it selfe, with the iudgement of your eies, &c.

A man of forty yeeres old cured by vnction, &c.

In the yéere of our Lord 1580. there came vnto me an other man being forty yéeres of age, which had a long time béene troubled with this great sicknes, and was diuers times in cure by diet, vnction and fumigation. He was infected in many places of his body: especially vpon his head were thrée mighty great nodes, which had corrupted the most part of all the whole substance of his scull through both the tables, as it is wel knowen to diuers Surgeons in this citie of London that haue séene the man, which by the foresaid vnction and other orders of this booke, was by me perfectly cured, &c.

A man, his wife, and three of his children cured by the vnction, &c.

In the yéere of our Lord 1582. I cured néere vnto the city of London, a man, his wife, and thrée of his children all at one time, and in one house, and within the space of sixe wéekes: the man and his wife were gréeued with this disease for the space of seuentéene yéeres, as they themselues confessed to me and diuers others, and had béene in cure oftentimes for the same, by diuers skilfull Surgeons beyond the seas, and also in England, but it profited them little: yet in the ende the Lord so

 prospered

prospered my labours, that they were by me perfectly cured with my vnction before nomitated, &c.

A Gentleman cured by the vnction, &c.

In the yeere of our Lord 1592. there was sent vnto me from Deepe in France, by a Physition and Surgeon somtimes dwelling in London, a very honest and skilfull man, a certaine Gentleman about the age of fiue and thirty yeeres infected with this disease called Lues Venerea, which sicknesse had continued vpon him some ten monthes with extreme paines, and diuers knots and hard swellings vpon his armes and legs, whereby his complexion and strength was greatly consumed and wasted: he was diuers times in cure (as he said) by the purging and drying diets, and also by minerall pils and potions, and other purgations: but in conclusion he found small helpe or amendment thereby, so he disliked these proceedings, and did confer with the foresaid Physition what was his best course to take. After much speech had togither, at the length they concluded, that without further staying, he should presently depart for England: at the length he came to London and inquired for me. After his arriuall, he conferred first with certaine Physitions and Surgeons, before I had any vnderstanding or knowledge of him, & the most of them caried a hard opinion against the vnctions, saying that the vnctions would make but an impefect cure, & spake against it most notorious and open vntruths, for in the end I healed him perfectly with this vnction following, with other ordinary remedies before spoken of,

The vnction.

℞. Axungiæ porcinæ lib.i.
Butyri recent. lib.ß.
Olei laurini
Hirundinum
Vulpini
Paralysi
Chamæmelini } ana.℥.i.
Masticheſ
Olibani } ana.℥.i.ß.
Theriacæ opt.
Spermatis ceti } ana.℥.ß.
Styracis liquidæ ℥.i.
Terebinthinæ Venet.℥.ij.
Argenti viui ℥.ii.ß.
Misce.

And here lastly to conclude, I do admonish the discret Reader, not to beleeue or credite the vaine folly or madnesse of some men, which so bitterly and maliciously speake against this vndoubted cure of vnctions, made with quicksiluer, sith it is confirmed by so many excellent men of great

great experience. Amongst the rest, I read of late a certain historie out of *Tagaltius*, noted as followeth. There was (saith he) a certaine begger, full of the French pocks, who for certaine daies lay couered all his body in horse dung, hauing no more than where to fetch his breath, for it was plaine stable dung, often moistened with horse pisse, and which putrified: he got by this practise, that he drew out all the venom: but it is further to be noted, that he added withall, an ointment made of bores grease and quicksiluer: neither kept he any other diet, than what his scrip gaue him, and yet by this meanes he was perfectly cured. Notwithstanding freendly Reader, I do not say, neither is it mine opinion, that the vnctions are to be vsed to all persons alike, nor at all times, but according to the cause, strength, and constitution of their bodies, &c. Neither would I haue any man of Art to be disswaded at the words, or writings of those men, who maliciously oppose themselues against this manner of cure by vnctions, and some of them principally do it for their lucre and gaine, to support their owne priuate practises and waies of curing, which themselues extoll aboue others, and not of any iust cause otherwise, as I haue often knowne by experience: and to say the truth, many of these finde-faults, are very ignorant in the order of curing by vnctions, vnlesse it be by reason of a little ordinary reading, which is truly compared and likened to him that is dismembred, and so he hath as it were but one leg to trust to, or hop on. And thus I end, with this breefe note of the curing the foresaid Gentleman, which was done and performed in the house of one *Isam*, dwelling at Dowgate in London, a place kept and ordained for the curing of such sicknesses and diseases, &c.

An historie.

Other very good Vnctions.

An other very good vnction. Arceus.

℞. Axungiæ porcinæ ℥.viij.
Butyri ℥.j.
Olei anethini
Chamæmelini
Laurini } ana.℥.ß.
Vnguenti dialthææ ℥.ß.
Argenti viui extincti cum succo limonum ℥.iij.
Et fiat linimentum, &c.

Another approoued Vnction.

Another vnction. Vigo.

℞. Olei Spicæ ℥.j.
Vnguenti pro spasmo ℥.ii.

Axungiæ porcinæ ℥.iiii.
Olibani ℥.ß.
Euphorbii ℥.i.ß.
Vnguenti dialthææ } ana.℥.i.
Vnguenti Agrippę }
Argenti viui ℥.iiii.extincti in aceto,& sputo hominis ieiuni.
Et fiat linimentum secundum artem.

Ambrose Pare, a very diligent and carefull man in the true studie and practise of the Art, saith, that it is very profitable and necessarie, that quicksiluer be first boiled in viniger, with sage, rosemary, time, cammomill and melilot, and after strained: and being farther moued with the like care, he doth say, that the best way to straine the quicksiluer is through a rams skin, for if it be pressed togither it doth pearce through it, and leaueth the filth and dregs in the inside of the skin, &c. and may then be mixed (as is before said) in the vnctions.

The order of making such necessarie vnguents and oiles, as are vsed in the vnctions, and so neere as I can, I will set downe euery authors name, as before I haue done: otherwise peraduenture some would say by me, as they haue said by others, that I haue decked my selfe with other birds feathers, or published in mine own name other mens trauels, &c. Cap. 9.

Vnguentum dialthææ compositum Nicolai.

Vnguentum dialthææ compositum Nicolai.

℞. Radicum althææ lib.ii.
Sem. lini } ana.lib.i.
Fænigræci }
Pulpæ scillæ ℥.vi.
Olei lib.iiii.
Ceræ lib.i.
Terebinthinæ ℥.ii.
Resinæ } ana.℥.vi.
Picis græcæ }

Let the rootes be chopped and brused with the seedes, and so stand three daies in 8. pintes of water, then boile them, & take two pounds of Mucilage, and boile it with other things till all the waterinesse be consumed, then

then adde thereto these gums following, Galbani, gummi hederæ, of ech ℥.ii. being first dissolued in wine viniger, &c.

Vnguentum martiatum paruum Nicolai

Vnguentum martiatum paruum. Nicolai.

℞. Fol. lauri lib. iii.
Rutæ lib.ii. ß.
Maioranæ lib.ii.
Rorismarini lib.i.ß.
Myrti lib.i.
Balsamitæ
Seminis ocymi } ana.℥.vi.
Butyri ℥.v.
Styracis
Medullæ ceruinæ
Adip. vrsini
Gallinacei } ana.℥.iiii.
Mastiches ℥.iiii.
Thuris ℥.ii.
Olei nardui ℥.i.ß.
Olei communis lib. vi.
Ceræ lib.iiii. Make hereof an vnguent according to Art, &c.

An vnguent called Vnguentum Vulpinum, which I haue many times vsed in the stead of Vnguentum Martiatum.

Vnguentum vulpinum.

Take a Fore, and draw out the entrales, then take Rosemarie, sage, iuniper leaues and berries, dill, wilde mariorame, and mariorame of the garden, lauender and camomill, of ech halfe a pound, stamp these herbs in a morter of stone very finely, and cut the fore in péeces, and put to the fore the foresaid herbes, so prepared in a faire vessell of eight gallons, and put to them fower pints of sallet oile, of oile of neates féete a pound, of calues suet, of déeres suet, of goose grease, of brocks grease, of ech halfe a pound, of sea water thrée quarts, and as much of good malmsey, set all these togither on the fire, & boile them till the wine and water be consumed, and that the flesh and bones be separated a sunder, that you may with a paire of tongs grabble out the bones from the rest, thus let it be taken off and pressed through a péece of canuas, and kéepe it to your vse. This is most pretious for lamenesse and aches, &c.

Vnguentum

Vnguentum Genistæ.

Vnguentum genistæ. M.Keble.

℞. Fol.Genistæ lib.vj.
Chamæmelini
Meliloti
Absinthij
Ebulij
Aparinis ligustici
Coronopi Ruellij } ana.m.ij.
Butyri recent.lib.j.

Beate all these togither, and put thereto Olei oliuarum lib.ji. let all these rot togither sixe weekes, then put to them
Vini albi lib.ij.
Ceræ citrinæ ℥.xij.
& fiat vnguentum.

I tooke this vnguent out of a written booke of secrets of my Masters, M. *George Keble*, and I haue approoued it profitable. Surely *Alexander* the great was neuer more bound to *Aristotle* his master for his lessons in philosophie, than I was bound to him, for giuing me the first light and entrance, into the knowledge of this noble art of Chirurgerie, &c.

Master Kebles ointment for aches, wherewith I haue found much profit by the vse thereof in my vnctions.

M.Kebles vnguent.

℞. Fol.saluiæ
Rutæ } ana.lib.j.
Fol.lauri
Chamæmeli
Absinthij } ana.lib. ß.
Adipis ouini lib.iij.
Olei oliuarum lib.iiij.
Vini albi lib.ij.

First chop the herbs small, and then bruse them in a morter, and chop the suet very fine, and beate all well togither vntill the suet be not séene, then take it forth, and put it into a faire vessell, and couer it close, and so let it stand the space of ten daies: then take it out of the vessell, and put it into a brasse pan, and then put in also the wine, and set it ouer a soft fire of coles, and let it boile gently till the wine be consumed, and that the herbes ware parched, then take it from the fire, and straine it, &c.

Vnguentum

Vnguentum Aregon Nicholai.

Vnguentum aregon Nicholai.

℞ Rorismarini
Maioranæ
Radicis ari
Serpilli
Rutæ
Rad.cucumer.Asinini } ana.℥.iiii.ß.
Fol.lauri
Saluiæ
Sabinæ } ana.℥.iii.
Pulicariæ maioris
Minoris } ana.℥.iiii.
Rad.Brioniæ ℥.iii.
Laureolæ ℥.ix.
Nepitæ ℥.vi.
Mastiches
Olibani } ana.ʒ.vii.
Pyrethri
Euphorbii
Zinziberis
Piperis } ana.℥.i.
Adipis vrsi
Olei laurini } ana.℥.iii.
Olei Moschelini ℥.ß.
Petrolei clari ℥.i.
Butyri ℥.iiii. aut quantum sufficit.
Olei lib.v.
Ceræ lib.i.℥.iiii.

The herbes and rootes must be gathered in May, and infused in the oile seauen daies, then boile them on the fire the space of two howers, and in the end straine them, and adde to the waxe, and so relent them togither, &c.

Vnguentum Agrippæ Regis.

Vnguentum Agrippæ regis.

℞. Rad.Brioniæ lib.ii.
Rad.cucumer.asinini lib.i.
Scillæ lib.ß.

Ireos

Ireos ℥.iii.
Rad. Filicis
Ebuli } ana. ℥.ii.
Tribulorum aquaticor.
Ceræ albissimæ ℥.xi.
Olei albissimi lib.iiii.

Let all these rootes be cut and brused, and infused in oile for the space of eight daies, then boile them againe at a gentle fire of coles the space of one hower, then straine them, and adde to the waxe, being cut in small peeces, and so relent them togither, & fiat vnguentum, &c.

An vnguent, which doth ease paines, and also resolueth and mollifieth hard swellings.

A resolutiue and mundificatiue vnguent.

℞. Mucilaginis seminis lini
Rad. althææ } ana. ℥.ii.
Olei spicati
Amygdalorum dulcium
Chamæmeli } ana. ℥.ii.
Gummi Arabici
Dragaganthi } ana. ʒ.ii.
Cum cera fiat vnguentum, &c.

Now followeth the order of making such oiles, as are vsed also in the vnctions.

Oleum Laurinum taken out of Gesnerus and Lanfranke.

Oleum Laurinum Gesneri & Lanfran.

℞. Bay berries finely broken, and infused sixe daies in wine, and then put them vp in bags, and draw out an oile by presse. The order of making this oile is also commended by *Rogerius*. Another order how to make the said oile, taken out of *Lanfranke*: Gather first your berries, and boile them in tribus libris vini, then straine out the liquor of the berries and wine, and put thereto olei lib. tres, letting it boile againe vntill the wine be consumed, then take it off the fire, and reserue it to your vse, &c.

Oleum Terebinthinæ taken out of Gesnerus.

Oleum Terebinthinę Gesneri.

℞. Of cleere turpentine, what quantitie you will, and for euery pound of turpentine put three ounces of the ashes of hard wood. I do vse in the stead of ashes the powder of tilestones, glasse or sand, which after the

the mixture togither, put all into a retort set on a furnace, and in the beginning distill it with a soft fire, untill all the moisture be drawen: after increase the heate with a stronger fire, untill all the oile be distilled and come, which keepe diligently in a glasse. This oile is the secret of *Gabriel Fallopius*.

Oleum Liliorum.

℞. Oleum Oliuarum dulc. what quantity you please, and put it into a faire strong glasse, and adde thereto of the flowers of Lillies being shred so much in quantity as conueniently will go into the glasse, so that they be alwaies couered with the oile: then set it in the sunne seuen or eight daies, and at the eight daies end, boile this in Balneo Mariæ fiue or sixe howers: then take it off, and let it coole, and straine it, and put to againe as many more fresh flowers, and this do three or fower times, as you may get the flowers from time to time. But note, that this last infusion must stand in the sunne a moneth or sixe weekes, before you put it into Balneum Mariæ, then being well boiled straine it, and reserue it to your use. After this maner and order I do make Oleum rosarum, chamæmelinum, anethinum, absinthinum, violarum, sambucinum, &c. and I find this order to be certaine and good in operation, &c. Oleum Liliorum. Clowes.

Oleum Chamæmelinum Pauli.

℞. Florum chamæmeli (demptis foliis albis) ℥.iiii. Olei oliuar. lib. ij.ß. the floures must be dried in the shadow fower and twenty howers, then put them with the oile into a glasse with a narrow mouth being well stopped, and let it stand in the sunne forty daies, &c. Oleum chamæmelinum Pauli.

Oleum Anethinum.

℞. Fol. & flor. anethi contus. ℥.iiij. Olei veteris lib.j. let these be also dried in the shadow, and make it in the like order, as you do the foresaid oile of Chamemill, &c. Oleum Anethinum.

Oleum rosarum completum Mesuei.

℞. Olei ex oliuis maturis in aqua fontana multoties loti quantum velles, put into this of red rose leaues so many as you thinke good and conuenient, set these in the sunne eight daies, then boile them in a double vessell one the fire three howers, then take new roses and do as Oleum rosarum complectum. Mesuei.

aforesaid, and do also the third time, and put the fourth part of water of the infusion of roses, and let it stand in the sunne fortie daies, then straine it again, and put to the iuice of roses, and after let it stand in the sunne, &c.

Oleum Lumbricorum.

Oleum lumbricorum.

℞. Lumbricorum terrestrium lib. ß. being sliced and washed in Vino albo, then take Olei rosf. Omphacini lib. ij. Vini albi ℥. ij. boile all these in a double vessell to the consumption of the wine, then straine it and reserue it to your vse, &c. Now héere I end this chapter of the making of certaine vnguents and oiles, which I daily vse in the vnctions, and come to the description of certaine approued diet drinks and purging potions, very profitable helpes also in this cure, &c.

Master *Gales* drying diet drinke, approoued most precious for the curing of diuers diseases, but specially for the disease called *Lues Venerea*, which good old man florished in our time, being an Englishman borne. He wrote certaine books of Surgery, specially an Institution, very plainly and distinctly for the benefit of all yoong students in Chirurgery. He was had in much reputation in the great warres of King *Henry* the eight, being then in France chiefe Surgeon in the English army, as in his writings it may more plainly appeere, yet it is not vnknowen to many, that some with despitefull fruitlesse bablings thrust foorth themselues in defacing, reiecting and contemning his painfull labours and skill, whose dealings therin are vncharitable, malicious and vndiscreete. Cap. 10.

M. Gales diet drinke.

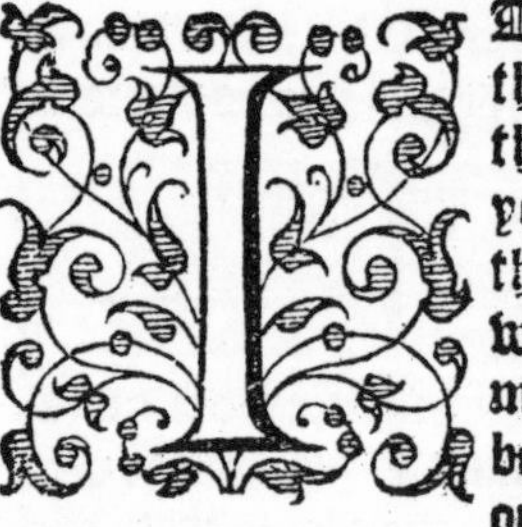

It is to be considered that there are thrée sorts of this wood, that is to say, that which is very old, that which is meane and old, and that which is yong, and the boughs of the trée, and euery one of these do differ in quality one from the other: that which is yong with the branches also is of a moist and more airy substance than the other two be, and that which is old is more hard of digestion, and slower in operation, and longer before any cure may be done with it: wherefore we do commonly vse that which

which is yong and whitest with the barke of the same, for it doth not dry away naturall moisture of mans body, so soone as the old doth: and that is by reason of his moistnes, yet in his property he doth as much as the other. The old and the black wood is good to make oiles and such like things, either by decoction or distillations, for it is more fat and gummy than the other is, except it be rotten, and then is not good in medicines. This wood hath a singular propertie against Chameleontiasin, and also against other moist and reumatike sicknesses, for it letteth putrifaction, and altereth the euil qualities of the humors, it comforteth the stomack, and openeth the obstructions of the liuer, and moueth the body to sweate, and helpeth nature to put forth many perilous and contagious vapours by the pores outwardly. Also that which is oldest being boiled in decoction, and other waies by Art prepared, is very good for vlcerations, fistulas, aches and paine, being applied according to the Art of Surgery, as is mentioned in this booke in diuers places.

And first of all to make the decoction to drinke inwardly, yée shall vse the yongest wood, or the branches with some part of the barke of the same, as it followeth héere,

The diet drinke of Guaiacan or the holy wood.

℞. A gallon of faire water, and put it into a new earthen pot, the which may hold thrée gallons of water, or two gallons and a halfe at the least, and put thereunto of the yongest wood aforesaid lib.j. with some of the barke in powder, licorise brused ℥.ij. séeth them vpon a few coles, the pot being close couered, that so little of the aire may passe away as is possible, and let it stand vntill it be very hot, then take it of the fire, and let it stand twelue howers, then boile it vpon a soft fire vntill the halfe be consumed, then straine it and put it in a faire vessell. This is the strong drinke which they may drinke of morning and euening, at ech time ℥.viij. and euery morning the sicke person to sweat after he hath taken of the same drinke by the space of two howers.

And for the second decoction which they must vse with their meat, you must put to the same wood that you strained from your first decoction, with so much water as you did before, and let it stand and stéep, as aforesaid, in the same pot by the space of twelue howers, and then boile it vntill the halfe be consumed, as you did the other before.

In weake bodies and cold we haue vsed to put into the first decoction, one pint of malmsey or sack, a little before that it be taken from the fire, and in the latter drinke we haue vsed to put in rackt Rhenish wine, but in strong bodies, and those that be not so weake, we must vse to giue it alone without wine. The bodies must be well prepared before they take this drinke, or enter into the rules of this diet, by the space of twelue or xiiij. daies, in the which those humors may be purged that do hurt the

 bodie,

bodie, or maintaine the disease: and then when the bodie is well purged, they may enter into the same diet, giuing them no other drinke, but the same abouesaid, and diminishing meate by little and little, vntill sixe daies be past: then let them haue so little meate as they may liue withall: for if they should take much meate, nature should be so occupied about the digestion of the same, that it should not be able to ouercome and digest the sicknes, or else such quantitie of humors might growe thereof, that might still maintaine the disease: yet neuertheles those that be cholerike bodies may take more meate and moister meates, than those that be flegmatike and moist bodies. Generally their meates must be rosted, and of good nourishment, and easie to digest: as mutton, veale, capons, rabbets, chickens, feasants, partriges, blacke birds, thrushes, and other small birds of the wood, this must be onely their meates, and rosted without salt, except in cholerike bodies that be like to fall into some feauer, they may haue their meates boiled, and eate them with a little veriuice.

In flegmatike bodies they may forbeare their supper, and hold them contented with one meale a day, except at night a few raisons of the sun, and blanched almonds: but cholerike bodies must haue some meate at night to satisfie their stomacke withall, bicause they will sooner digest it, for they haue no such quantitie of moist humors, as the flegmatike or sanguine person hath.

Their bread must be onely bisket, made with a few anise seedes and sugar without salt: they may take of this bread more or lesse, according to the strength of their stomacks and complexion, as it afore said.

This diet or order must be kept by the space of forty or fifty daies more or lesse, according to the necessitie of the sicknes: and euery sixth day the body must be purged with some gentle medicine meete for the disease, and for the complexion of the man. That day that they take their purgation they may not drinke their drinke, nor sweate in the morning, nor no time that day: all other daies they must sweate, for sweating is the chiefest matter that is required in this maner of cure. They must vse also other maner of necessary things, as sleeping, quietnes, company, and conuenient place, and aboue all things to be kept close in all the time of the cure, least that the aire might enter in and stop the pores, and let them to sweate, & do other displeasures. This maner of curing is most praised of many of our late writers, and cheefly of *Hutten* a German, *Nicholas Massa, Iohan. Baptista, Montanus, Antonius Gallus, Alfonsius Ferrens, Anthonius Musa, Michael Bologenis, Leonardus Fuchsius, Iohannes Tagaltius, Dominicus Leanus Luensis,* and many mo, which were very long heere to reherse, they haue written all in the commendations of the wood, but in in effect they haue concluded in the vsing of it, as I haue made mention heere aboue, and I my selfe haue found great profit, and gotten great credit thereby. I inuented my selfe a syrup, which I made with the same decoction strongly boiled, vntill it come to a syrup: with the which syrup I did great cures, and chiefly when the patient was very weak, as ye shall finde by the triall, *Finis T.Gale.*

Calmetheus purging potion for Lues Venerea.

Calmetheus purging potion for Lues Venerea.

℞. Ligni sancti lib.j.
Cortic.eiusdem lib.ß.
Aquæ purissimæ lib.x.

Infuse them, and let them soke xxiiij.howers, and boile them to the consumption of the third part, then take

Radicum Enulæ campanæ } ana.℥.ß.
Dactylorum ab ossibus separatorum }
Senæ orientalis ℥.j.

Steepe them in Vini albi lib.vj. fower and twenty howers vpon the hot imbers, so that the wine be almost ready to seeth, then straine it, and put that first decoction to this, and adde Sacchari lib.ß. Cinnamomi ℥.j. and fower howers after let the patient take fiue or sixe ounces before supper, and when he goeth to bed as much, and put to the residence of the first decoction Aquæ purissimæ lib.xv. and boile it to the consumption of the third part, and put to as much sugar and cinnamon, as is sufficient to make it pleasant to drinke.

Another.

D.Hectors purging potion for Lues Venerea.

℞ Pul.guaiaci ℥.x.
Cortic.eiusdem } ana.℥.ij.
Zarzæ parillæ }
Cardui benedicti }
Herbæ paralysis } ana.m.ij.
Agrimonij }
Hermodact. ʒ.ij.
Turpeti ʒ.iij.
Agarici ʒ.ij.
Zinzib. ℈.iiij.
Rhabar.opt. ʒ.iiij.
Fol.Senæ orient.℥.iij.
Calami aromat. ʒ.ij.

Infuse

Infuse these fower and twenty howers in faire running water lib. 20. then let it be boiled in Balneo Neptuni or Mariæ, to the consumption of the third part and somwhat more: in the end of the boiling put in of Cinnamon ℥.ß. being first brused, and so let it stand till it be cold, then straine it, and reserue it to your vse. The dose to be taken at a time is sixe or eight ounces, according as the patients stomacke and strength is able to beare it. This foresaid drinke is of great importance for the curing of Lues Venerea, the first manifest proofe thereof I saw experienced by the author himselfe, and since I haue many times approued it, and also found great profit thereby, &c.

Another, D. Ludford.

D. Ludfords purging posion for Lues Venerea.

℞ Ligni sancti ℥.xij.
Corticis eiusdem ℥.ij.
Senæ ℥.iiii.
Colocynth. ℥.ß.
Cinnamomi ℥.i.
Passularum sol. ℥.iiii.
Glycyrrhizæ ℥.ii.
Ceruisiæ lib.xvi.

Boile these to the consumation of the third part.

Another decoction, or purging diet drinke.

Another purging potion for Lues Venerea.

℞. Ligni sancti ℥.xii.
Cortic. eiusdem lib.i.
Senæ ℥.iiii.
Zarzæ parillæ ℥ iiii.
Colocynth. ℥.ß.
Vini albi lib.xvi.
Ceruisię fortis lib.viii.

Boile these also to the consumption of the third part, as is before said.

M. Bakers purging potion for Lues Venerea.

M. Bakers purging potion for Lues Venerea.

℞. Ligni guaiaci lib.ß.
Corticis eiusdem ℥.iiii.
Zarzæ parillæ ℥.iii.
Cardui benedic. }
Lupul. polytrici } ana. m.i

Capil.

Capil. Veneris
Asplenii } ana. m. i.
Fol. senæ ℥. iiii.
Polypodii querc. ℥. iii.
Seminis anisi & feniculi ana. ℥. ß.
Glycyrrhizæ ℥. ß.

Infuse these for the space of fower and twenty houres, in Aquæ communis lib. xii. then let it boile untill the consumption of one halfe, then adde to your Senæ, and let it stand in the embers for the space of six houres after, and then straine it, and of this let him drinke morning and evening, the quantitie of six ounces at a time, or more if neede be, at the discretion of the giver, for the space of one and twentie daies: if you boile it in Balneo Mariæ, it will be the better, &c.

Another most rare and singular decoction, or purging diet drinke, for the cure of Lues Venerea, comming with extreme aches, which drinke I obtained of Doctor Randole, by great friendship and intreaty, &c.

D. Randols purging potion for Lues Venerea.

℞. Limaturæ guaiaci ℥. vi.
Zarzæ parillæ ℥. iiii.
Corticis guaici
Rad. Helenii sicci } ana. ℥. i. ß.
Rad. & fol. verbasculi
Fol. card. bened.
Rad. iridis viridis
Sem. anisi
Fæniculi
Petroselini } ana. ℥. i.
Succi verbasculi ℥. iii.
Senæ Alex. ℥. iii.
Polypodii
Agarici
Trochis. } ana. ℥. i. ß.
Hermodact. ℥. ii.
Colocynth.
Stœchados } ana. ʒ. iiii.
Mechoacæ
Rad. asari } ana. ʒ. vi.
Rad. fœn.
petroselini } ana. ℥. iiii.

Glycyrrhyræ

Glycyrrhizæ
Vuar um paſſ.rub. } ana.℥.iiii.
Ficuum inciſarum numero x.

Infundantur omnia in lib.xvi. Ceruiſiæ fort.lup. per xxiiij. horas coqu. ad dimid. ante finem ebull.adde

The ſecond decoction.

Bugloſſæ
Boraginis
Violarum
Capil.
Anthos } ana.m.ß.

Et cum ſaccharo albo, dulcorentur doſ.℥.viii.vel vi.mane tantum, ceruiſiæ fort. lup.lib. xvi.coq. ad lib.viii. cum prędict.ingredientibus, quibus adde bugl.borag.viol.cap. ven.anthos ana.m.ß. & cum ſacchar. dulcorentur: ſeruetur pro ſecundario potu, &c.

A note of certaine trochiſces or perfumes, well approued for the cure of Lues Venerea, which order and way of curing, hath been a long time practiſed by men of learning and great experience. Cap.11.

The cure by trochiſces or perfumes.

It is to be noted, that theſe kinde of trochiſces or perfumes following, are not commonly vſed, except ye haue firſt approued all the foreſaid waies of curing to be in vaine. Neither is it to be practiſed of any man, which hath not had long practiſe and experience in this order of curing by trochiſces: prouided allwaies, that the bodie be firſt well prepared, and purged according to the order afore deſcribed: and then may this way of cure be orderly done vnder a canapie, or a pauilion, in the middeſt thereof ſhall be placed a ſtoole with a round hole in the middle, like to a cloſe ſtoole of eaſement, whereon the patient ſhall ſit naked, to receiue the fume, and there muſt alſo be left a fit place, in ſome one part of the pauilion, to receiue aire, & take breath as often as cauſe requireth, and let there be put vnder the foreſaid ſtoole, a chaſing diſh of coales, wherein you ſhall caſt in the trocheſces, and ſo let him or hir there ſweate one houre or two, as his ſtrength wil ſerue, and let him be conueied to his bed with ſpeed, being orderly lapped in a warme ſheete, forgetting not that his bed be very well warmed with a warming pan, and

and there also let him sweate, if he can one hower or two, and then after rest, untill the next day, eschewing colde and aire, as much as is possible: the second day he shall receiue the trochisces or perfumes againe, as he did the day before, and so the third and fourth day, untill the flux of flegmatike matter doth orderly rise, and then be very carefull for the curing and preseruing of their mouthes, with such gargarismes, syrups, lotions, & other needfull remedies (afore published in the cure by unctions) as well in dieting as otherwise, which do also serue necessarily for the curing by trochisces: and for that I haue well approued these trochisces following to be very profitable in this cure, I haue thought it good to publish the same, and to prefer them before any others that I haue yet knowne, &c.

Trochisci Vigonis.

℞. Cinnabrii ℥. ii.
Thuris
Styracis liquidæ } ana. ʒ. i. ß.
Fiant Trochisci.

Another.

Trochisci. Clowes.

℞. Cinnabrii ℥. ß.
Beniam.
Styracis calamitæ
Myrrhæ
Rad. ireos Florentinæ
Masticḥes
Olibani } ana. ℥. ß.
Nucis muscatæ
Maceris } ana. ʒ. iii.
Theriacæ ʒ. ii.
Terebinthinæ q. s.
Fiant trochisci.

Another.

Trochisci Ander. Matth.

℞. Cinnabrii ℥. iii.
Myrrhæ
Thuris } ana. ℥. i.
Aloes hepat.
Sandarachæ
Styracis calamitæ
Beniam. } ana. ʒ. iii.
Fiant trochisci.

Another.

Frendly Reader, I haue in all my seueral practises, obseruations and experiments, béen very carefull to publish those speciall remedies, which by cōtinual exercise & long experience haue ben wel approued. Amongst others, this fume here following, for the cure of Lues Venerea is greatly commended, and faithfully deliuered vnto me by M. *Gerard*, a man well practised and experimented in the Art of surgerie, and also of profound knowledge and iudgement in the nature of herbs and plants,

℞. Lapidis hematitis, Cinabrii, ana. partes æquales.
Misce.

Another.

Trochisci Ambros. Par.

℞. Cinnabrii ʒ.i.
Beniam., Myrrhæ, Styracis, Opoponacis, Olibani, ana. ʒ.ß.
Masticℏes, Macis, Thuris, ana. ʒ.ii.

Let them be made into trochisces with turpentine, and so vse them as is before said.

Another.

Trochisci. I.P.

℞. Myrrhæ, Mastiches, Beniam., Styracis calamitę, ana. ʒ.ii.
Antimonii crudi ʒ.ii.
Cinnabrii ʒ.i.ß.
Styracis liquidæ ʒ.i.
Fiant trochisci.

Some also do vse to minister these fumes and such like, in the bed, in a chaffing dish of coles, hauing ordained in a readinesse a stole or frame fit for the chafing dish to stand in, and so to beare vp the clothes, and somtimes it is to be placed betwéene the patients legs, or other wise, as they sée occasion, onely to receiue the fume: when he hath so sweat,

as

as is aforesaid, abate the clothes by degrees, and let the patient coole gently, and thus procéed with the rest of the cure in the same maner and order, which I haue héere in this booke truly set down. To conclude this maner and order of curing by fumigations, and héerein then I thought it not amisse to note vnto the freindly Reader, that a few yéeres past, their repared vnto me a certaine man infected with Lues Venerea as followeth. He had first a stinking Gonorrhea and running of the reines, and therewithall corrupt bloody matter continually flowing, which as I gathered by relation of the patient, precéeded from the glandula called prostata, which sharpe and venemous matter did excoriate the condit of the yard in certain places, but most specially vnder Glans, by meanes héereof, he was wonderfuly tormented in the making of his water, and likewise in the erection of his yard. Moreouer a little before he came vnto me, he had two Venereous buboes of ech side of his groine one, which for want of good looking to, went in againe of themselues, and so neuer came to suppuration, with some breakings out and ache in the night. To come vnto my principall purpose, he earnestly desired me to tell him truly what his griefe might be, I answered him secretly to his question proposed, that it came of a naughty venemous matter: what meane you by that said he? I pray you speake plainly and openly, for here are none but these two gentlemen my good freinds: It is a spice of the french disease said I: Nay that is not so (sir) by your leaue, as cunning as your are, for I haue shewed my water to certaine Physitions, and they can find no such thing, but onely an inuoluntarie flux, or loosenesse of the reines called Gonorrhea: I told him the water will hardly shew that disease, though the body be very greatly infected, and so I referred my iudgement héerein to the learned, and to them that haue knowledge: Well said he if it be so, I pray you tell me how I should come by it? No man (said I) can tell that better than your owne selfe: but mine opinion is: if I be not deceiued, by some common harlot. That cannot be true neither said he, for she whose company I do vse and frequent, I will be sworne is constant onely to me. I answered he might easilie be deceiued, for it is a common and true saying, She that will be a whore with one man, will no doubt be the same with another if oportunitie serue. Then he departed, being greatly disquieted in mind, and said, he would aske further counsell, and come to me againe. But as it was reported by one of his friends, he went presently to mistris honestie his swéete hart, and began to looke discontented vpon hir, and after told hir that one had said, he was infected with the great disease, and that he got it by some ill woman, the which to heare caused hir to shed many a dissembling teare, and desired him for the loue she had borne to him a

An historie.

long time, that he would not put vp such an iniurious slander at their hands, that had so reported of hir, sith it touched hir credit greatly, and she did sweare vnto him, but onely for him and hir husband she was as good a maid as she was borne of hir mother. But the gentleman was wiser than to satisfie the bloody minde of a harlot, and after by perswasions of his friends went downe into the countrie where he dwelt, to seeke helpe for his disease, neuertheles God prospered not their labours that tooke him in cure: for within xij. moneths after, he returned againe to London, for further helpe of his disease, which was in that time and space so confirmed, that being seene of diuers skilfull physitions and Surgeons in London, who refused to deale with him: in the end he came againe to me, and when I saw him I knew him not, neither by his fauour nor by his speech: Why (said he) do you not know me: Truly sir (said I) you must pardon me, I haue forgotten you. Then he told me certaine true tokens aboue named, which I very well remembred, then after other talke had, he shewed me the roofe of his mouth, which was pearsed through with corruption of the bone, and many sharpe and putrified humors continually distilling from the braine, by meanes whereof he had but an vnperfect voice, and very hardly could be vnderstood any word he spake. Also he was still troubled with Gonorrhea fœtida, and his body greatly pined and wasted, as it were in a lingring consumption: in the end he desired me to take pity vpon him, otherwise his disease did threaten his vtter shame and ouerthrow, but he trusted I was the man that could make him whole, and as for money I should not want. Truly I did in my hart and minde greatly bewaile his miserie, and so told him plainly he was now past my cure, and therefore I would in no wise deale with him. So very sorrowfully he departed from me: but shortly after one tooke him in hand, and warranted to cure him perfectly for a large summe of money, and that within the space of seuen weekes, and did administer vnto him his fume, which (as it was reported) he receiued the smoke thereof chiefly in at his mouth, being in his bed sitting vpright, and a cloke or mantle cast ouer his head, and other clothes to keepe in the smoke or fume. At the second perfuming suddenly his head was taken with a conuulsion, and a maruellous shaking and trembling ouer all his body, and so he died. Truly this bold perfumer may very well be compared vnto him, that did vndertake and also warrant for a large summe of mony, to make an Asse speake within the space of seuen yeeres: which thing being knowen, he was greatly reproued, for that he did presume to do or vndertake such an impossible matter: He answered boldly, I am well assured to do & perform that I haue promised: for before that time appointed being seuen yeeres space, either he that

As good a maide as Malkins mare.

that laid the wager with me, or else the Asse, or I my selfe shall be dead and thus I shall be certaine and sure to saue my credit, and also gaine the money, and win the wager. I will héere leaue to speake any further of this dangerous enterprise and most vnfortunate experience, onely I do aduertise all students in surgerie, neuer to be too forward in warranting any thing, and to take héede that you do not vnaduisedly administer these trochisces or perfumes, bicause of the euill vapours of the brimstone and quicksiluer, whereof it is said the Cinnabrium is made, &c.

A dangerous enterprise, & a most vnfortunate experience.

Turbith Minerall is also said to be singular good in the cure of Lues Venerea. Cap. 12.

Take Quicksiluer oftentimes washed in viniger, and salt six parts, and let them be mixed with one part of the purest and finest gold, the gold being first melted in a crucible, and when it beginneth to waxe cold, adde vnto it the quicksiluer, being made hot in another crucible, & so mix it well togither, then adde vnto it so much Aquæ fortis, as will dissolue the gold, and make ther of a precipitate, this kind of Turbith is prepared with great pains, & it serueth for the collicke, quartans, & for Lues Venerea, and it requireth a time & charges, but being made, it ought to be put in a glasse vessell, and so to be set in the embers: & when it hath continued a time, whereby the strong water may euaporate forth by force of the fire, then it is become precipitate. But if you will make Turbith, then you must wash it well, and do it according to Art. But before you administer this Turbith mineral, let the patient be first purged with some good purgation, méete to purge this sicknesse: yet if the body be very foule, as most commonly it is, let blood also the next day: if the patient be strong, giue him xiiij. graines of this turbith mineral, & rowle it vp in Butyri recentis q.s. and make one pill and gild it. But remember before they take the pill, that they drinke a good draught of mutton broth, and at euery time they do vomit, giue presently some posset ale, mixed well with sugar. And thus you shall take thrée of these pils togither, hauing a day respit betwéene, according as the strength of the sicke patient will serue, and for healing of their mouthes, take posset ale, and mixe with it honie of roses, and if the mouth grow foule, and furred, put to the iniection so many drops of oile of sulphur as will make it tart, and also to heale it vp, with some other good lotion, if néede so require, &c.

Turbith minerall.

Mercurie

Mercurie Diaphoreticum, a singular secret in the cure of Lues Venerea.

Mercurie Diaphoreticum. C. F.

℞. Mercurie that is coagulated with Lime ℥.i. rub it into fine powder, put it into a golden dish, or for want thereof, they say a dish made of good double glasse may serue the turne, let your dish stand in vineger almost to the brim, then put the spirit of wine vpon the Mercurie, & set it on the fire, and let it boile cleane away, then rub your Mercurie againe in fine powder, and put it into the dish againe, then adde more spirits of wine vpō it, as before: do this so oftentimes vntil you haue spent a quart of the spirits of wine, & after reserue it for a singular secret. I leaue the vse hereof to the learned Physitions, and those that are of daily experience with such kinde of remedies. My freends that gaue me these two secrets, did earnestly desire me, that I would promise them not to publish these remedies, or to make them common to all men. But after I heard them and other men being of great iudgement and skill, report them to be such rare and pretious iewels, in the cure of Lues Venerea, then I thought with my selfe, if they were a thousand times better than they are, I would here publish them for the good of other, which daily I know are troubled with the said disease, where all helpes that may be had, are oftentimes scarse able to serue their turne: no not amongst the best practised Physitions and Surgeons, the disease of his owne proper nature is so euill, &c.

In anno 1593. there came vnto me a gentlemans seruant, belonging to his husbandry, being a man of a sluggish or gullish nature, about the age of 30. yeeres, and of a very bad constitution of bodie, in complexion & colour like vnto a tawny Moore: he was infected with two great impostemes, in Inguina, called Bubones Venerei, of ech side of his flanke one, and vpon Glans and Præputium a number of foule and filthy warts, & withal the running of the reines, (which as he said) was the first begining of this euil. So after I had taken him in cure, & prepared him a lodging somwhat neere vnto my house, thē the first thing I did, I went about to ripē or suppurate his impostumes, therunto I applied for the space of 6. dais, a singular good maturatiue plaister, published in my former book, but it was not of that force to bring them to suppuration: then other sixe daies I continued with plaisters of Galbanum, and this also did him but small pleasure: after I had well considered, that this was but a hard beginning, I hoped of better successe, by the administring of this pultis following, ℞. Garlike and onions being rosted, of ech ℥.iij. of figs lib. ß. being boiled in a pint of malmsey, till all the wine be consumed: let all these be well beaten togither, then adde thereunto, of hard or stone hony ℥. iiij. the yelkes of fower egs, being hard rosted, the fat of restie bacon, lib ß. the oiles of camomill and lillies, of ech two ounces, the mucilage of the rootes of marsh mallows, fenigreeke, and lineseed, being made with white wine and water ℥. iiij. of sharpe and sower leauen, made of sower houshold bread, lib. ß. of beane meale, ℥. iiij. of saffron, ʒ. ß. make hereof a poultis according to Art. By the vse of this poultis within the space of nine daies, his impostumes were ripe and in state, and then they were opened by the common ruptorie or causticke: after all were opened, and the eschars remooued, I found a great quantitie of spungeous and corrupt flesh, and the humors that flowed, were like vnto bucke ly, and the more I mundified them, the fowler they were: also I did applie vnto the warts aforesaid, this powder following, wherwith I haue cured many, but it preuailed little with this patient, nor any thing else whatsoeuer, vntill I vsed the causticke stone, wherewith I did take most of them away: but by that time the eschars were remooued, the warts and spungeous flesh was growne againe. The said powder is this that followeth,

℞. Auri pigmenti
Sulphuris
Calcis viui } ana. ℥. ß.
Sabinæ ʒ. j.
Misce, & fiat pul. secundum artem, &c.

After I had thus continued for a space, and saw a small amendment, then I conferred with a very skilful physition, & imparted vnto him the course that I had taken about this cure: then he aduised me to giue him for certaine daies this purging potion, wherewith he said he had cured diuers that were greatly infected with Morbus Gallicus,

℞. Aquæ fontanæ lib. v.
Ligni sancti ℥. iiij.
Cortic. eiusdem ℥. ij.
Zarzæ parillæ ℥. iiij.

Let these be steeped fower and twenty howers in water being close couered, then set it on a fire of coles to boile gently, and when it is boiled neere halfe away, then adde to the rest

Sarsafras ℥. j.
Rhabar. opt. ʒ j.
Agarici ʒ. j.
Senæ orientalis ℥. j. ß.
Rad. Enulæ campanæ ℥. j.
Rad. Eringij ℥. j.

Sem.

Sem. anisi
Fœniculi } ana. ℥. j.
Petroselini
Passularum sol. m. j.
Vini albi lib. ij.

Let all these boile togither very gently one hower, and then take it off the fire, and let it stand till it be cold, then straine it, and drinke a good draught heereof in the morning, and another at two of the clocke in the after noone, and another when he goeth to bed. But you must also, when you haue strained the strong drinke, fill your pot with the like quantitie of water againe, and put it into the old stuffe, and let it seethe as you did the other drinke, till halfe be sodden away, then straine it, and drinke it at your dinner and supper. Ye shall heere note, that I continued this drinke till he grew weary of it, and said he should be discredited, and lose his seruice if he continued long in this cure. I must confesse, so long as I vsed this drinke his greefes did come faire, and he amended reasonably well: but when I left it off, all did fly out again: then I forthwith gaue him xiiij. graines of Turbith minerall, (as is before said) but it wrought not to my liking: the next time I gaue him xviij. graines, and that wrought to good effect: the third time I gaue him xviij. graines more, the which pils brought him to a good flure at the mouth, which was cured, as it is before specified: by meanes heerof he was made whole of his impostumes, and also of all the rest of his greefes, within the space of xiiij. daies, and so continueth still.

The discription of certain approoued remedies by me collected, which are very needfull and necessary helps in this cure: and I haue gleaned them thus togither, like the poore Bee which gathereth hir hony from euery sweete flower.

Cap. 13.

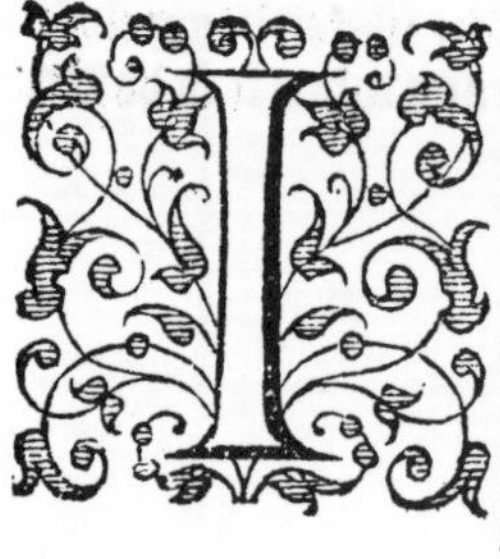

I Haue thought it not amisse heere to adioine certaine other approoued remedies, which I haue found to be very conuenient for the cure of this sicknes, & also for the curing of wounds, vlcers, & apostumes, & for that in some persons which are greatly infected with sharpe and gnawing humors, that do eate and exulcerate the parts affected, & being of long continuance it falleth out thereby often and many times, as I haue before said.

said, some to haue virulent, corrosiue and malignant vlcers, fraudulent and deceitfull vlcers, with hard callous and swolne lips and edges: and other some to haue corrupt, putrified and rotten vlcers, which become foule and filthy with great losse of substance, which must be againe restored, and sometimes vlcers and nodes with corruption of the bones in diuers parts of the body, so that these maladies haue néed of such remedies héereafter described, before ye can safely and orderly administer the vnctions or fumigations: for by these remedies, those vlcers before named are greatly corrected of their malignitie, and the hard tumors and knottie swellings are to be opened with caustick medicines, when they will not yéeld to mollification or resolution. And when they be clensed and purged from annoiances aforesaid, which wil conueniently be done by these remedies following, then may yée safely vse the vnctions or trochisces, and cure perfectly this disease by the order which is before described, &c.

Ceratum Vigonis cum Mercurio.

Ceratum Vigonis cum Mercurio.

℞. Oleor. Chamæmel.
Anethin.
Spicæ
Lilior. } ana. ℥. ij.
de Croco ℥. i.
Pinguedinis porcinæ lib. j.
Pinguedinis vituli lib. ß.
Euphorb. ʒ. v.
Thuris ʒ. x.
Olei laurini ℥. j. ß.
Ranarum viuentium num. vj.
Pinguedinis viperæ ℥. ii. ß.
Or in sted thereof I do put in
Ex pinguedine hominis ℥. ii. ß.
Lumbricorum lotorum cum vino ℥. iii. ß.
Succi radicum ebuli
Et enulæ } ana. ℥. ii.
Squinanti
Stæchados
Matricari } ana. m. i.
Vini odoriferi lib. ii.

Let them séeth al togither vntill the wine be consumed, then straine them, and put to the straining Lithargyrii lib. i. Terebinthinæ ℥. ii. make a cerote with sufficient white waxe after the maner of a sparadrop,

drop, adding in the end of the decoction Styracis liquidæ ℥.i.ß. then take the cerote from the fire, and stir it vntill it be luke warme, and afterward put thereunto Argenti viui cum saliua extincti ℥.iiii. and stir it about well vntill the quicksiluer be incorporated, Et fiat ceratum.

Another.

Another cerot. Clowes.

℞. Emp. de meliloto Mesuei ℥.vi.
Emp. diachylon Magni Mesuei ℥.iiii.
Emp. oxycrocei descriptione Nicolai ℥.ii.

Relent all these plaisters with an easie fire of coles, and in the cooling yée shall put in of my vnction, or some other good vnction ℥.ii. or ℥.iii. and stir it well vntill it be colde, ye may spread this cerote either vpon leather or vpon linnen cloth, and so applie it, &c.

Another.

Another cerot. Botallus.

℞. Axungiæ porc. vet. lib.i. being cleane picked from the skins.
Pingued. gallinæ ℥.iii.
Olei de Terebint. ℥.ii.ß.
Euphorbii, Castorei — ana. ʒ.iii.
Styracis calamitæ ℥.i.ß.
Cinnabrii ℥.ii.ß.
Ceræ q.s.

To make it in forme of a cerot, in the end adde to it of quicksiluer very well killed ℥.iii. mixe all these togither, and worke it well vntill the whole masse be cold, bicause that which is heauy may not sinke to the bottome, &c,

Another.

Another cerot.

℞. Oleo. Liliace., Amygdal. dul., Medul. Cruris cerui — ana. ℥.ii.ß.
Mucilag. sem. lini, Fænigræci & althææ — ana. ℥.i.
Ceræ q.s.
Misce.

A plaister good for aches and paines, practised by M. Keble, and he called it his plaister.

A spiced plaister. M. Keble.

℞. Ceræ ℥.xii.
Resinæ ℥.viii.
Picis ℥.i.ß.
Olibani ℥.iiii.
Resinæ pini lib.i.
Adipis ceruini ℥.ii.
Croci ʒ.ii.
Maceris } ana.℥.ß.
Gariophyllorum }
Vini rub.lib.ii.
Misce & fiat emplastrum.

Emplastrum Oxycroceum descriptione Nicolai.

Emplastrum oxycroceum descriptione Nicolai.

℞. Ceræ }
Picis nigræ } ana.℥.iiii.
Picis græcæ }
Croci }
Terebinthinæ }
Galbani }
Hammoniaci } ana.℥.i.ʒ.iii.
Myrrhæ }
Thuris }
Mastiches }

Dissolue the Hammoniack and Galbanum in a sufficient quantity of viniger vpon a few embers vntill the viniger be consumed, then ad therunto your pitch, wax, rosin, and turpentine being melted togither, then put to your Mirrhe, mastick, and frankinsence being made in fine powder, continually stirring them togither till they come to the thicknes of a cerot: after you haue taken it from the fire, put in your saffron and make it according to Art. I haue proued this plaister to be a very good helpe in this sicknes being dissolued with these two plaisters following, according as I haue before specified, &c.

Emplastrum de Meliloto Mesuei.

℞. Meliloti ℥.vj.

Emplastrum de meliloto Mesuei.

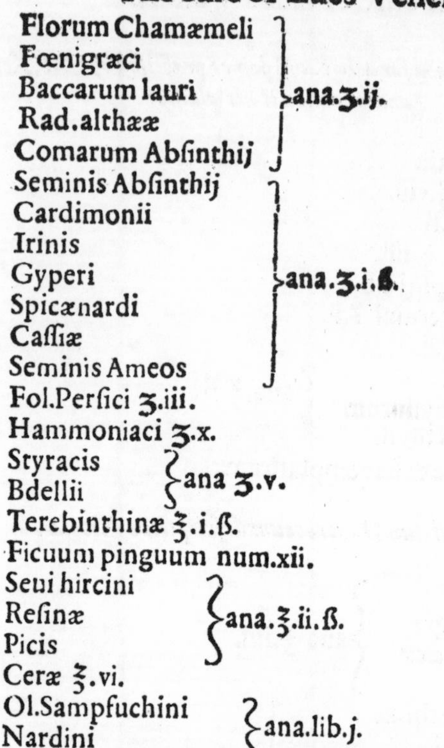

Florum Chamæmeli
Fœnigræci
Baccarum lauri
Rad. althææ
Comarum Absinthij } ana. ʒ. ij.
Seminis Absinthij
Cardimonii
Irinis
Gyperi
Spicænardi
Cassiæ
Seminis Ameos } ana. ʒ. i. ß.
Fol. Persici ʒ. iii.
Hammoniaci ʒ. x.
Styracis
Bdellii } ana ʒ. v.
Terebinthinæ ℥. i. ß.
Ficuum pinguum num. xii.
Seui hircini
Resinæ
Picis } ana. ℥. ii. ß.
Ceræ ℥. vi.
Ol. Sampfuchini
Nardini } ana. lib. j.

Boile your Melilot, Fenigræke and Camomill unto the consumption of halfe, then straine them, and put thereto the other parcels finely made into powder: and boile them againe, adding the oiles, turpentine and gums dissolued in vineger, then put to the rootes and figs being well brused, and wel boiled togither, and so make a plaister according to art.

It doth mollifie all hardnesses of the stomacke, liuer, splene and other intrals, it doth also cease vehement dolour and paine, and healeth the windines of Hypocondria.

Emplastrum Diachylon magnum Mesuei.

Emplastrum diachylon magnum Mesuei.

℞. Lithargyrij lib. j.
Oleor. Chamæmelin.
Irin.
Anethin. } ana. ℥. viij.
Mucilag. sem. Lini
Fœnigræci } ana. ℥. xii.

Althææ

Althææ
Ficuum pinguium } ana. ℥. xij.
Vuarum passarum
Succi iridis
Scillæ æsypi } ana. ℥. xij. ß.
Ichthyocollæ
Resinæ pini } ana. ℥. ij.
Ceræ flauæ
Fiat ceratum vt prius.

It doth digest and mollifie all hardnesses, and therefore may with great profit be applied vnto Scirrus, and other hard tumors, &c.

A speciall good resolutiue and maturatiue plaister.

A very good resolutiue and maturatiue plaister. Clowes.

℞. Oleorum Irin.
Liliace. } ana. ℥. iij
Ceræ citrinæ lib. j.
Resinæ lib. j.
Resinæ pini lib. ß.
Picis albi ℥. vj.
Galbani ℥. ij.
Gummi Ammoniaci ℥. iiij.
Opoponacis ℥. ij.
Croci ʒ. j.

Dissolue your gums in malmsey or muscadell, and make thereof a plaister according to art. If you haue not the oile of the flower deluce, then take the whole quantitie of the oile of lillies, and you shall finde this plaister to be a rare and worthie secret, &c.

A plaister against inueterate vlcers.

F. Rassius.

℞. Emplastri de Cerusa optime cocti lib. ß.
Mercurii extincti in aqua vitæ ℥. iii.
Fiat emplastrum bonæ constitutionis secund. artem.

Emplastrum Epispatices, ad omnes juncturarum dolores ex frigiditate, Odolpius Occo.

Emplastrum epispatices, Odolpius Occo.

℞. Ceræ veteris
Colophiniæ } ana. lib. i.
Resinæ pinæ

Calcis

Calcis viuæ
Aluminis plumati } ana.℥.i.
Arcenici

Relent your ware and rosin with a small quantitie of oile, then strain in your powders being finely powdered, and mire with them Aceti fortis q.s. boile all togither at a gentle fire to the forme of a plaister.

Emplastrum Triapharmacum Mesuei.

Emplastrum triapharmacum Mesuei.

℞. Lithargyrii subtilissime triti } ana.lib.i.
Aceti vini
Olei veteris lib.ii.
Et fiant emplastrum secundum artem.

Emplastrum Ceruse, Gale.

Emplastrum cerusæ, Gale.

℞. Olei Ros.lib.ij.
Axungiæ lotæ in aquæ rosaciæ & vini lib.i.
Cerusæ subtiliss.lib.iiii.
Ceræ albæ ℥.viii.

Let these be boiled gently togither ouer a soft fire of coles, stirring them continually untill they come to the substance of a plaister.

Emplastrum desiccatiuum, a very commodious plaister deuised by Master Iohn Hall Chirurgion of Maidstone in Kent : a man very studious and laborious in writing diuers bookes in the English toong, chiefly for Lanfranks briefe surgerie, the which he hath most kindly commended to posteritie, as a testimonie of the loue he bare vnto his natiue countrie and common wealth, wherein somtimes he liued.

Emplastrum desiccatiuum. I.Hall.

℞. Lapidis calaminaris ℥.viii.
Terræ sigillatæ ℥.iiii.
Cerusæ ℥.iiii.
Lithargyrii auri & } ana.℥.ii.
Argenti
Boli Armeniæ ℥.i.
Lithargyrii plumbi ℥.ii.
Sanguinis draconis ℥.ß.
Terebinthinæ ℥.vi.

Seui

Seui hircini } ana.lib.i.
Ceræ }
Et fiat emplastrum.

Mundifiyng or abstersiue vnguents.

Vnguentum mundificatiuum.

Vnguentum mundificatiuum.

℞. Resinæ ℥.viii.
Colophoniæ ℥.iiii.
Ceræ lib.i.
Gummi Opoponacis } ana.℥.i.
Eruginis æris }

Relent your waxe, oile, suet, and rosin all togither, then straine the gum, being first dissolued in vineger, and boile it a little vpon a gentle fire of coles, then take it of, and so put in your viridis æris in fine powder.

Another mundifiyng vnguent.

Another mundifiyng vnguent.

℞. Gummi Ammoniaci ℥.ii.
Bdellii }
Olibani } ana.℥.i.ß.
Aristolochiæ }
Sarcocollæ }
Myrrhæ } ana.℥.i.
Galbani }
Lythargyrii ℥.iii.
Aloes } ana.℥.i.
Opoponacis }
Viridis æris ℥.ß.
Resinæ pini ℥.iii.

Dissolue your gums in vineger, and powder the rest, then adde thereunto Ceræ citrinæ lib.i. Olei communis lib.ii. & fiat vnguentum.

Another mundifiyng vnguent good for the vlcers of Lues Venerea, Clowes.

Another mundifieng vnguent. Clowes.

℞. Vnguenti viridis ℥.viii.
Vnguenti popul. compos. ℥.ii.
Pulueris Mastiches ℥.i.
Mercurii præcipitati ʒ. ii.

Labour all these in a morter, and after reserue it to your vse.

Other

Other more strong mundifiyng vnguents, very necessary in subduing spungious flesh in the aforesaid corrupt and filthy vlcers.

Vnguentum Ægyptiacum Mesuei.

Vnguentum Egypriacum Mesuei.

℞. Æruginis æris ℥.v.
Mellis optimi ℥.xiiij.
Aceti fortis ℥.vii.

Boile these to the thicknes of hony.

Another of the same.

Another of the same.

℞. Mellis lib.ii.
Viridis æris ℥.iiii.
Aluminis rochæ ℥.iii.
Aceti lib.i.

Boile this as the other, &c.

Another of the same.

Another of the same.

℞. Mellis rof. lib.ii.
Aquæ vitæ } ana.lib.ß.
Aceti vini albi }
Viridis æris ℥.ii.
Vitrioli albi ℥.ii.

Let your Viride æs be made in fine powder, and mix all togither, and boile it as afore said, to the thicknes of hony: it doth not onely mundifie and clense foule and filthy vlcers, but also scaleth corrupt & rotten bones.

Heere followeth potentiall cauteries, or caustické medicines, which do take away superfluous and rotten flesh, and also do open, or breake great nodes, hard tumors or swellings, when they do not yeeld to other good medicines, seruing for resolutions, mollifications, or suppurations, and also for the speedie discouering of corrupt and rotten bones, and for making of large issues in the head, armes, and legs, or in any other parts of the body, hauing great care vnto the veines, arteries, sinewes, and such like parts.

Ambrose Pare his caustické stone.

Ambrose Pare his caustick stone which he bought.

A speciall good caustick stone, which *Ambrose Pare* chiefe chirurgeon vnto the French king hath published, and saith, if it be applied to the

arme

arme in quantitie of a pease, for the space of halfe an houre, that it doth eate away the skin, and the flesh that is vnder it, euen vnto the bone, without paine, especially if the part it selfe be without paine and inflammation, and it maketh an vlcer as big as ones thombe, and it leaueth an eschar so soft and moist, that it will easily fall away within fower or fiue daies, without scarification, and it is thus made,

The description of it with others of a certaine Alchymist, and he calleth it his silken or veluet cauterie.

℞. The stalks or stems of beanes, burne them to ashes, and take of the ashes of oken wood well burned thrée pound, let them be infused in halfe a paile full of running water, let them be stirred often in a cauldron, then adde thereto of vnslackt lime lib.iiii. which being extinguished, let all that be stirred togither diligently for the space of two whole daies, wherby the lie may be the stronger, then let it be strained through a thicke and grosse linnen cloth, and receiued from the strainer in a bason, and so poured thrée or fower times on the ashes, that the ly may endue it selfe the more easily with a firy facultie: afterwards let it boile in a Barbars bason, or in an earthen pot well leaded, ouer a quick fire of liue coles, vntill it become thicke: but in the measure and maner of thickning, a great part of the secret or Art doth consist, for that the ly being made thicke, & congealed into salt, ought not to stand so long ouer the burning coles, vntill all the liquor do vanish away, being consumed by the scorching heate of the fire, for so the power of the forenamed medicine, which doth consist in the vapors, should vanish away also: therefore before that it come vnto the extreme drinesse, it must be taken from the fire, that is to say, then when there is yet some of the thicke liquor remaining, which may not hinder this cauterie to be made, as you list, and to retaine their forme receiued in making, when these cauteries are made, they must be kept in a thicke glasse, closely stopped, least that the aire should come to them, for then they would melt, and therefore it is good to set them in a close and warme place, &c.

Another causticke stone, which M. Fr̄auncis Rassius, one of the french kings Chirurgeons did giue vnto me, &c.

℞. Aquæ lib.xxx.
Fæcis vini vsti lib.iii.
Calcis viui lib.vi.
Cineris querci &
Caulium fabarum } ana.q.s.

Another caustick stone.

F. Rassius.

Let all these lie infused in the water twelue houres in an earthen vessell, being strong and well nealed, then giue it a walme at the fire, and let it rest fower and twenty houres til it be very cleere, then let it be well strained through a cotton strainer, and so boile it with a fire of coles untill it come to the forme of a stone, then breake it in small peeces, or great peeces, as you thinke best. The older this causticke stone is, the lesse paine it causeth, as master *Rassius* saith, &c.

Another caustick or ruptory.

The ordinary causticke or ruptory.

℞. Lixiuij saponarii lib. i. Calcis viui q.s. as will bring it to the forme of an unguent. But before you boile it let the Calx viua be made into very fine powder, then boile it very gently that the Calx may mixe well with the Lixiuium, and if it be too thick put in more of the Lixiuium, stirring it often with an iron spatula, and so boile it again gently til it come to the forme aforesaid.

This caustick or ruptory you may spread as you please upon pledgets of lint or tow, as you do any unguent, and so apply it with discretion: this caustick worketh not without paine, neuerthelesse ye shall finde it a very good one, although it seeme but simple, and made without curiositie, &c.

Vnguentum incarnatiuum.

Vnguentum incarnatiuum

℞. Resinæ, Ceræ citrinæ ana. lib. ß.
Terebinthinæ ℥. iiij.
Olibani, Mastiches ana. ℥. j.
Myrrhæ, Sarcocol. ana. ʒ. iij. ß.
Olei mast., Mellis ros. colati ana. ℥. j.
Farinæ hordei ℥. ij.
Misce, & fiat vnguentum.

Another.

Another. G. Keble.

℞. Olei ros. ℥. xii.
Resinæ ℥. xii.
Ceræ citrinæ ℥. viii.
Terebinthinæ ℥. vi.
Mastiches ℥. ii.

Oliban

Olibani ℥.iiii.
Croci ʒ.ii.
Misce,& fiat vnguentum,&c.

Vnguentum Basilicon.

℞. Olei comm.lib.i.ß. Vnguentum Basilicon.
Ceræ } ana lib.ß.
Resinæ }
Picis naualis lib.i.
Adipis vaccini ℥.viii.
Terebinthinæ ℥.iiii.
Ouorum luteorum numero iiii.
Misce,& fiat vnguentum secundum artem.

Vnguentum sanatiuum.

℞. Olei comm. } ana. lib.j. Vnguentum sanatiuum.
Resinæ }
Ceræ citrinæ lib.ß.
Adipis ouini lib.ß.
Terebinthinæ ℥.xij.
Lapidis calaminaris lib.j.
Misce,& fiat vnguentum secundum artem.

Another.

℞. Terræ sigillatæ } Another.
Lapidis calaminaris } ana.℥.iiij.
Lithargyrij auri }
Olei communis lib.j.
Ceræ ℥.xij.
Camphoræ ʒ.j.
Misce,& fiat vnguentum secundum artem.

Vnguentum desiccatiuum rubrum.

℞. Lapidis calam. } ana.℥.iiij. Vnguentum desiccatiuum rubrum.
Terræ sigill. rub. }
Lithargyrij auri } ana.℥.iij.
Cerus. }

Ceræ ℥.v.
Camph. ʒ.j.
Olei ros.& Violar. } ana.℥.vi.

Melt the waxe and the oile, and when they be neere cold, strow in the powders, and stir them with a spatula, and in the end put in the Camphor dissolued in oile of roses q.s.& fiat.

Vnguentum Diapompholygos Weckeri.

Vnguentum diapompholygos Weck.

℞. Olei rosati
Ceræ albæ } ana.ʒ.vi.
Succi solani ʒ.i.
Cerusæ lotæ ʒ.ii.
Plumbi vsti & loti
Tutiæ præparatæ } ana. ʒ.i.
Thuris ℥.ß.
Misce, & fiat vnguentum secundum artem.

Vnguentum Catapsoras very profitable for itch, scabs, tetters, or ringwormes, &c.

Vnguentum Catapsoras. D.Hill.

℞. Cerusæ lotæ in aqua plantaginis & aceti ℥.iiij.
Myrrhæ
Thuris } ana.ʒ.iiii.
Sanguinis hirci ℥.j.
Chalciteos ʒ.ii.
Plumbi vsti ʒ.j.
Lithargyrij ʒ.iij.
Lapidis calaminaris ʒ.iij.
Mercurij sublimat. ʒ.i.
Succi plantaginis &
Semperuiui
Oleorum Violarum &
Nymphææ } ana. ℥.ii.
Axungiæ porcinæ lib.ii.
Misce, & fiat vnguentum secundum artem.

An vngent good for the hemorrhoids. G.Keble.

An vnguent good for the Hemorrhoids.

℞. Vnguenti ros. ℥.ii.
Vnguentum populei comm. ℥.i.ß.

Vitellorum

Vitellorum ouorum num.i.
Opii ʒ.ß.
Misce.

A Cataplasma, which doth resolue and also suppurate hard tumors or swellings.

℞. Farinæ triticeæ } ana.ʒ.i.
Farinæ fabarum
Farinæ sem.lini } ana.ʒ.vi.
Farinæ Fœnigræci
Ficuum contusarum ℥.i.ß.
Axungiæ veteris ℥.ii.
Croci ℈.i.
Vitellorum ouorum num.ii.
Fiant cataplosma.

A Cataplasma to resolue & suppurate. Andernacus.

Another Cataplasma of the same operation.

℞. Rad. Liliorum & } ana.m.i.
Althææ
Florum Mal.
Ficuum pinguium num.viii.
Coquantur in hydromel, then adde to
Sem. Lini & } ana.℥.i.
Fœnigræci
Farinæ hordei ℥.ii.
Olei Liliorum ℥.i.
Axungiæ porcinæ ℥.i.ß.
Et fiat cataplasma, &c.

Another. A.Parry.

A good water to stay the speading of eating or corroding vlcers, comming of Lues Venerea, being in the mouth, throte, or yard.

℞. a quart of running water, two faire orenges being good and full of iuice, and cut asunder in the middle, one good roote of Enula campana, being somwhat more than an ounce, and being sliced in two péeces, then boile all these till halfe be wasted, in an earthen pot being well nealed or glassed, then straine it, and put the liquor into the pot againe, and adde to it two drams of Mercury sublimat, and boile it a little, and then reserue it to your vse, &c.

A very good Mercurie water obtained of a friend.

A

A good water called Aqua viridis, very profitable for vlcers on the yard.

Aqua viridis.

℞. Aquæ cælestis lib. viii.
Sacchari Candi lib. j.
Viridis æris ℥. iiii.

Boile these togither, and in the end put in the Viride æs, &c.

Another water to cure vlcers and excoriations in the vrinarie passages.

A water to cure vlcers and excoriations in the vrinarie passages.

℞. Aquæ rosarum & Solani } ana. lib. i.
Agrimonii m. i.
Sacchari Candi ℥. ii.
Floris æris ℈. i. ß.

Boile all these till almost halfe be consumed, then ad to the infusion, of roses ℥. ij. then straine it, and reserue it to your vse, &c.

Another cooling and drying water for vlcers in the condit of the yard.

Another good water for vlcers within the condit of the yard.

℞. Aquæ plantaginis ℥. iiii.
Aquæ rosarum ℥. ii.
Aquæ hord. ℥. viii.
Syr. ros. ℥. ii.
Collyrii albi sine opio ʒ. i. ß.

A very good iniection to appease paine, and also coole and heale vlcers, and excoriations in the vrinarie passages.

A very good iniection to appease pain, and also it doth coole and heale vlcers and excoriations in the vrinarie passages. I.M.

℞. Lithargyrii auri, Ceruss. Venet. } ana. ℥. iiii.
Camphoræ ℥. ß.

Make al these into fine powder, and then take ℥. ii. of this powder, and put it into a pint of white wine, and when you will vse it, a little before shake the glasse well and warme it, and then iniect it into the yarde, and when the wine is all spent, then may you put vpon the ingredients as much more fresh wine, &c.

Another

Another good water of great operation, for the consuming and wasting away of hard tumors and nodes, and ceasing of extreme and raging paines, comming of Lues Venerea, by me approoued, and also ratified and confirmed by men of great experience, &c.

A very good water of great operation, for curing of raging pains, & consuming of nodes and hard swellings, &c.

℞. Caryophillorum } ana. ℥. ß.
Pyrethri }
Euphorbii } ana. ʒ. ii.
Piperis longi }
Gingiberis }
Croci orient. }
Cerusæ } ana. ʒ. vi.
Aluminis }
Sulphuris } ana. ℥. ß. ʒ. j.
Salis nitri }
Cantharidarum } ana. ʒ. iii.
Cardamonii }
Theriacæ Andromachi ʒ. v.
Mercurii sublimati ℥. ii.
Vini sublimati lib. ii.
Misce.

The maner and order of apping this water is thus: there must be made a small smooth sticke, three or fower inches in length and in compasse, (as it were) like vnto a swans quill vpon the one end. The top of the sticke shall be tied and fastened on with a strong thred, a peece of linnen cloth wrapped, or doubled round about the said end of the sticke, like vnto a painters pensill, the which you shall dip in the said water, and so minister or applie it onely vpon the parts agreeued, and not otherwise, be it either vpon nodes, or vpon other parts of the body, as the ioints, &c. During all which time you do dip or wet the greeued parts, you must hold very neere therevnto a chafing dish of coles, that this water may the better drie in, and do this so many times vntill it blister the skin, then staie your hand, and leaue of the vse of the said water, vntill the blistered parts haue run wel, and so suffer them to heale vp again of themselues, and then begin againe as aboue said. And vse this maner and order, so many times vntill the pains be taken away, and the nodes or hard swellings cleane consumed. Some haue thought it good to applie vpon the parts blistered, colewort leaues, being annointed with sweete butter: then for the curing of the accidentes of the mouth, which fall out by by reason of the applying of the said water, you shall safely cure the same with those remedies which before I haue published in this booke, &c.

A water good to cure Vlcers in any part of the body.

A water good to cure vlcers in any part of the body. H.O.

℞. Arg. viui
Aquę fortis } ana.℥.i.

Put these togither in a glasse, and let it so stand two daies, but often shaking it, till it be congealed.

Herb. chelidoniæ
Solatri
Ruthæ } ana.m.ß.
Fol. rof. rub.℥.ß.
Aristolochiæ rotund.℥.i.

Boile all these herbes in a pottle of water, untill halfe be consumed, then straine it, and take of this water, and of the congealed Mercury, & mixe it togither, according as you will haue it strong, and so keepe it for your use.

The composition of a most singular water, with the excellent vertues of the same, deuised by my master, M. George Keble practitioner both in Physicke and Surgerie.

℞. Aniseedes lib.i.
Licoris lib.ß.
Cinnamon ℥.ii.
Galingale
Ginger
Orras roots
Enula campana
Stichædos
Fenell seedes
Caroway seedes
Olibanum and
Mastiches } ana.℥.i.
Nutmegs
Graines
Cubebs
Cloues
Commin seedes } ana.℥.i.

Amonum

Amonum ſeedes Ameos ſeedes Pionie ſeedes Baſill ſeedes Winter Sauorie Sweet Marieram ſeedes	ana.℥.j.

If you haue not theſe ſeedes, you may dry the herbs, and take of ech m.j.

Chamæpitys m.ß.
The berries of Iuniper ℥.ij.

Long Pepper Calamus Spikenard Maces	ana.ʒ.iij.

Setwall ʒ.j.
The rootes of Angelica ℥.ß.
Cypris ℥.iiij.
Ligni Aloes ℥.ß.
The rootes of Alchanet ℥.j.
Strong Ale or Malmſey iiij.gallons.
Sugar ℥.iiij.

Put the Sugar and the Alchanet rootes into the receiuer, &c.

This water is ſaid to be good for thoſe that haue their ſinewes ſo drawne, that they cannot ſtand vpright, and for all paſſions that procéede of melancholie and cold: it is alſo approoued good for aches, and eaſeth the gowt: and to be giuen inwardly, it breaketh the ſtone, and is moſt excellent for colde and weake ſtomacks, and it comforteth ſuch as ware faint in the cure of this ſicknes, and is alſo good for other diſeaſes, which I héere omit.

The maner and order of ſearing and preſeruing dead bodies for a long time.

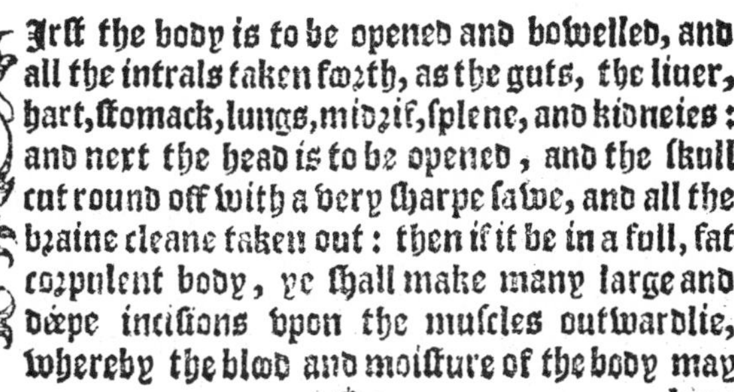

Irſt the body is to be opened and bowelled, and all the intrals taken forth, as the guts, the liuer, hart, ſtomack, lungs, midrif, ſplene, and kidneies: and next the head is to be opened, and the ſkull cut round off with a very ſharpe ſawe, and all the braine cleane taken out: then if it be in a full, fat corpulent body, ye ſhall make many large and déepe inciſions vpon the muſcles outwardlie, whereby the blood and moiſture of the body may

In leane bodies you may omit your inciſions, or ſections outwardly.

haue the better and freer passage to issue or come forth, then let all the parts of the body both inwardly and outwardly be washed with verie strong viniger, and after let it be well dried with a spunge. But if it be the will and pleasure of the friends of the dead, to haue the body preserued and kept for any long time and space, bicause many being of high calling, and so require an honourable buriall. Then yée shall fill the belly, head, and all the cuts or incisions outwardly with this powder following, or such like which hereafter shall be set downe,

The powder. Clowes.

℞. Calcis viui extincti
Pulueris baccar. lauri &
Sem. cumini
Cyperi
Ireos
Origani
Absinthii
Lauend.
Rosar.
Nucis muscatæ
Cariophylli } ana. q. s.

I haue also with good successe in meane persons filled the cauities and ventricles before named, onely with Calx viuum extinct. without any other addition, all which performed and done, the dissections are presently to be very closely sowed vp, to the intent the powders do not fall out againe, then the body is to be rowled and made vp orderly with this seare cloth or some other as you shall thinke best: which maner of rowling aforesaid, may better be learned by sight & experience, than by any mens writings otherwise. But I say if the body is to be preserued any long time before it may be buried, then vse the more double of seare cloth, to som twelue double, to other som sixtéene double, & some twenty double, more or lesse, as you sée occasion for a longer or shorter time.

The seare cloth. Clowes.

℞. Ceræ citrinæ lib. xii.
Resinæ lib. 50.
Seui ouini lib. vi.
Picis albæ
Resinæ pini } ana. lib. iiii.
Olei petrolei vel de spica q. s.
Misce & fiat secundum artem.

Which done let the body be leaded, and very well & close sodered, and after put into a coffin of wood being orderly pitched and seared, then put into the coffin some swéete powders, and let there be no fire in the roome where the body is placed, neither any great resort of people, for I know that

that hurt may come thereby. I haue by this maner and order of preseruing, kept a body very swéet without leading or coffining aboue two moneths, being in the hottest time of the summer. Some men of greater knowledge and experience, as *Vigo* and others, do first of al administer a sharpe clister made of viniger and salt water, wherein Myrrha, coloquintida, salt and alum hath béene sodden, &c. But my selfe neuer yet vsed so to do, if the body were presently to be bowelled, but forthwith followed my order before rehearsed. Also *Vigo* commended this powder, and willeth that the body be filled therewith. R. Flocks, or shauings of cloth diet with graine or some other cloth, with as much of these powders, braied salt, alume, of ech thrée parts, of cloues, nutmegs, cinamon, al the sanders, fräkinsence, myrrhe, Terra sigillata, of euery one of them one part, of nep, Serpillum, rosemary, coriander, wormwood, roses, and mirtils, of euery one a hanfull and a halfe, stamp these togither and bring them to powder, and then he willeth all the body to be wrapped in this sparadrop, R. Black pitch, rosin of the pine, Colophinia, frankinsence, mastick, storar, gum arabick, dragagant, melt these at the fire, and make héereof a sparadrop, &c. Moreouer he also willeth to ad to this sparadrop certaine powders, as those of his before named or such other. *Ambrose Pare* likewise commendeth these odoriferous powders, wherewith the body is to be filled,

Vigo his clister.

Vigo his powder.

Vigo his sparaprop or seare cloth.

Amb. Pare his powder.

Puluer. rosar.
Chamo.
Melil.
Balsami
Menthæ
Anethi
Saluiæ
Lauend.
Rorismar.
Maioran. } q.s.
Thimi
Absinth.
Cyperi
Calami aromatici
Gentianæ
Ireos Florent.
Assæ odoratæ
Caryophil.
Nucis muscatæ
Cinnamomi

 Styracis

Styracis calamitæ
Benioini
Myrrhæ
Aloes
Santal. omnium } ana.q.s.

Now heere to make it further knowen unto all yong students in Surgery, and others which are fauourers of this noble Art, and all good Artists, that it hath beene oftentimes signified unto me by diuers Gentlemen, Physitions, & Surgeons, specially by master *G. Baker* one of hir Maiesties Chirurgeons, of the excellency and great skill of M. *Ambrose Pare*: amongst many matters, this one thing I noted, which is worthie to be admired, that he had at his house in Paris the body of a condemned man, who being executed and dead, he begged it of the Judge or Judges, the which after he preserued and kept uncorrupt and sound for the space of twenty yeeres and more, in such sort, that a man might behold, see, and handle all the muscles of one side of his body, which he had cut off by the heads, and so hanged downe seuerally one by another, and that which is most strange, the lungs also, the hart, midrife, stomacke, melt and raines he also preserued and kept. And the haires of his head and beard, and nailes he did often cut, and yet they haue grown out againe, remaining whole and sound: it is said his maner of preseruing dead bodies is first to macerate and dip the body being bowelled, and pricked full of holes in the flesh, in a Tub full of strong vineger, and of the decoction of bitter things, as of Aloes, Rue, Wormwood, and Colocynthid, and so let it lie therin for the space of twenty daies, putting thereto eleuen or twelue pound of Aqua vitæ, and then set them upon their feete in some warme and dry place, &c. After this maner it is reported, the Aegyptians use to preserue their dead bodies for a long time, and being first so seasoned, it is thought a body may be preserued as it were for euer.

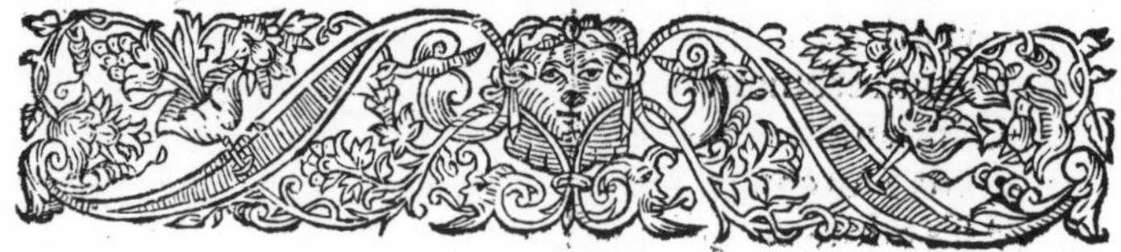

An admonition to the friendly Reader, in defence of publishing this Booke.

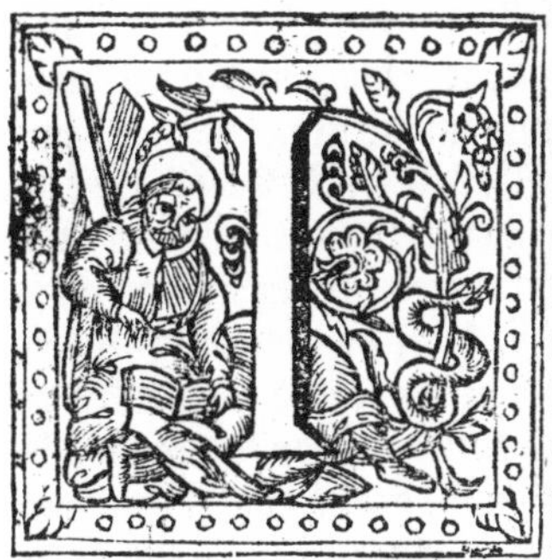

Haue heeretofore said, there is no booke so profitable for matter, or so pleasant for penning, which hath not had from time to time some that haue misliked it in both parts, not onely backbiters and whisperers, but also such as will seeme to saie somwhat, least they should be suspected to know little or nothing, who haue not sticked to set themselues as it were in a despitefull and mortal hatred, against many profitable works, which being a thing sufficiently knowne to all of any reasonable capacitie, no man needeth then to maruell, though against so simple a Treatise, & so obscure a writer, there rise vp many (not men of learning and iudgement in the Art) whose reprehensions I shall most willingly accept of: but some such that either in malice vnto the man, or for lacke of vpright iudgement in the matter, or bicause they enuie the light of knowledge in others, in respect of their owne praises, and vaine liking of themselues, haue many times both priuately & openly offered themselues to the disgrace of this poore treatise, & haue plainly said, they do dislike not only this booke, but also other works of Physicke or Surgerie, that should be penned in the English tong: vnnaturall men in my iudgement, enuying the good of our countrey and common wealth. It imbaseth the Art (they say) & maketh it too common, whereby euery bad man and lewde woman is become a Surgeon: and thus it is a hinderance to a number of good and honest Artists, and that the benefit which commeth by reason of publishing books in English, doth not encounter or answer the discommoditie and hurt it bringeth with it: and therefore though it be lawful, yet it is not necessary to publish bookes of Surgery in English. But if I might be so bold to enter a little farther into this discourse, without offence vnto such angrie saints, which haue oftentimes shot a number of these malitious thunderbolts against many good men, for publishing books of Physicke and Surgerie in English, and moreouer they are so insolent and proudly minded, that they disdaine and thinke it a great indignitie vnto their persons, to read any booke of Physicke or Surgerie in the English tong: and forsooth, being demanded their reasons why, they haue saide they could easily proue it without a syllogisme. But to speake farther of their cauilling speeches so vnreproouable, I maruell

maruell why it is more vnfit for vs, that be true naturall English men borne, to publish bookes of Physicke and Surgerie in English, than for al other countrey men, to put forth their works in their own language. They haue said, bicause it maketh the Art too common, truly a reason of such wise men, very weakely vnderpropped, for this I know full well, that Art commeth to no man by succession, but by great paines, long studie, much care and diligence, and I am also full well assured, that one good Surgeon, is worth a number of such euill tonged persons, notwithstanding the boasting and bragging of their only skils: and moreouer the great helpes themselues vaunt they haue by their deepe knowledge in the varietie of tongs, which indeed being also ioyned with the like vnderstanding in the Art, is to be accounted no doubt a double benefit, or else not. Neuerthelesse, I trust they will grant that *Hippocrates* and *Galen* were men of great learning and also experience, who wrote many worthy bookes of Physicke and Surgerie in the Greeke tong, were therefore all those Grecians then Physitians, and Chirurgians, that did read their bookes? *Auicen* wrote in the Arabian tong: *Plinie* wrote many learned and worthy bookes in Latine, it was his owne naturall tong, were all those men also Physitions and Chirurgeons, that could speake Latine and read their bookes? I doubt it very much: for *Hippocrates* in his first Aphorisme saith: Mans life is short, the Art is long, iudgement is hard, and experience is deceitfull. If this Aphorisme be true, as I make no question it is, how then can euerie bad man, and lewd woman as they terme them, become Physitions and Surgeons in a short time, onely by reading of a fewe bookes of Physicke and Surgerie in the English tong? *Ambrose Pare*, a man of great diligence, and manifold experience in Surgery, saith, that man which hath not a long time been trained vp in the works of Art, nor hath not greatly frequented the lectures of learned doctors, but doth esteeme and boast himself to be a noble surgeõ, only bicause he hath read many books, is far deceiued, and there is no truth in him: If this wil not satisfie these malitious men, who are flatterers of many, and louers of few, vnlesse it be such as are like vnto themselues, who suppose the Art is so easie to be attained, as though it would presently fall into mens mouthes: let them I say read or inquire, how many excellent men haue writtẽ in French, of all sorts of Arts being their owne naturall tong: and likewise the Germanes, and other Dutch, very famous learned men: and many good men haue written sundry kinde of learned works in English, their naturall language, all which as I take it, haue had this generall purpose, to benefit their countrey and countrimen, which professe the Art, with part of that knowledge and vertuous labors, wherewith God

hath

hath blessed them in their seueral sciences, that their knowledge should not die with themselues, but remaine vnto posteritie, as a testimonie of their loue, to further the trauels of such as should follow them. Likewise *Cicero* saith, that we are not borne onely to benefit our selues, but our countrey, parents and freends: all which reasons, haue moued many good men, as master *Ambrose Pare*, to publish for the good of his countrey and common wealth in France, that excellent booke of Surgerie, which he painfully collected. But since it pleased God, he hath giuen place vnto time, and liueth we all hope, immortall amongst the heauenly ioies. Now they say, he was a man vnfurnished of the sacred gifts of Grammar & Rhetoricke, neither had he euer tasted of the sweet fountaine and welspring of Philosophie, and therefore could not be a good surgeon: he answereth such like cauillers, and telleth them plainly, that it is possible for a man to be a good Surgeon, although he had neuer a toong in his head. And if it be their pleasures to speake iustly and truly of him, he neuer went about to teach the toongs, but to write and teach the Art of Surgerie in the French toong vnto all yoong practisers, for the better releefe and comfort of many sicke and diseased persons. Howbeit, it is in vaine to contend with such kinde of persons, whose bitter words are like bitter corrosiues, but this is well knowne to be Morbus inueteratus, proceeding from a malitious, cankered, and poisoned stomacke, which I thinke is vnpossible euer to be cured: notwithstanding this worthy man, was well knowne to haue had a notable wit, and of a profound experience, seldom out of practise in the wars, oftentimes frequented the hospitals, and many learned lectures, and for his excellent iudgement, he was commonly called to consultations and conferences with the best learned Phisitions and Surgeons, and very well knowne to be excellently read, and learned in his Art: by reason whereof he was called to be the first and chiefest principall Chirurgeon vnto diuers kings in France for many yeeres, which could neuer haue beene without some great & worthy desarts in him. To conclude these my former speeches, with the graue and wise sayings of M. *Gale* our good countriman late deceased, and yet within the compasse of our memory, in what toong soeuer a man may get knowledge, the toong serueth not further but for the learning of the Art. Which foresaid reasons induced many other of our good countrimen to publish diuers profitable works of Physicke and Chirurgerie in English, as namely D. *Record*, D. *Phare*, D. *Turner*, D. *Langton*, D. *Bourd*, D. *Bailey* late one of hir Maiesties Physitions, D. *Bright*, with many other worthy Phisitions and Surgeon, as master *Baker*, one of hir Maiesties chirurgeons, master *Hall*, M. *Banister*, M. *Iemeny*, &c. What shall we thinke of that worthy knight sir *Thomas*

Eliot,

Eliot, of master *Trehiron*, of master *Lite*, of master *Barrowe*, of master *Bullen*, of master *Kellaway*, and such other worthie gentlemen: shall all their knowledge, all their painfull labours, and all their commendable works haue no better recompence, but a malitious vpbraiding, bicause they are penned in English? O wicked and spitefull minded men, vnworthy the benefit of so good labors, not vnlike in nature to the Cuckow, which deuoureth the birde that brought hir vp. These causes cōsidered, I hope I shall haue the lesse reason to be dismaid at the scandalous and vnkind reproches, foule ingratitudes & vaingloriious flouts and frumps of these immodest persons aforesaid, who behinde my backe in scoffing sort, haue derided these my paines & trauels: being indéed so many degrées inferior vnto these excellent men, whose learned works could not escape their cankered venemous throtes: and therefore séeing my principal purpose hath béen common with these famous men, that haue labored by their writings to farther the knowledge of the Art in our language, and that I haue taken part of the labor, though my gifts, and the fruits of my trauell be far inferior vnto them, I shall be content in like maner, to take part with them of the churlish gripes of this venemous broode, who bicause they haue forgotten, that they haue receiued their skils by the help of others, which went before them, are vnwilling to leaue behinde themselues, any profitable helpe for their posteritie. Thus much I haue thought good to write briefly against that vaine cauill of publishing bookes in English, séeing that héerin I deserue no more blame than those excellent men, which by their famous writings in their owne language, haue purchased themselues immortall thanks of all men that succéede them, &c.

Finis William Clowes.

If faults good Reader, heer do chance to pas,
As in my former books, I must confesse there was,
To my great greefe, and Printers discontent,
Such is our lot, we can it not preuent.

WILLIAM GODORVS SERGEANT Chirurgion vnto hir Maiestie.

I Needes must count Apelles wise,
VVhich was no doubt a skilful man,
That did not trust his owne deuise,
But would haue others iudge and scan,
VVhat was amisse, and what was well,
VVhereby he made his worke excell,

Yet did not he amend the shooe,
Vpon the Tailors fault he found,
For then should he but so vndooe,
The worke that was both good and sound,
But if a Cripple said he hault,
The Painter mended foote and fault.

So he that painfully hath pend,
This skilfull booke of Surgerie,
I needes must praise and eke defend,
Both worke and workman woorthily,
For men of learning, skill, and fame,
Far passing me, commends the same.

So what exceptions Tailors takes,
Againg the shooe, it shall not skill,
Or men vnlearnd that enuie makes
Against this booke to beare ill will.
I GODORVS do the same commend,
And wish him well, and so I end.

FINIS.

Ff

The nature and propertie of Quickſiluer, by G.Baker one of hir Maieſties Chirurgions.

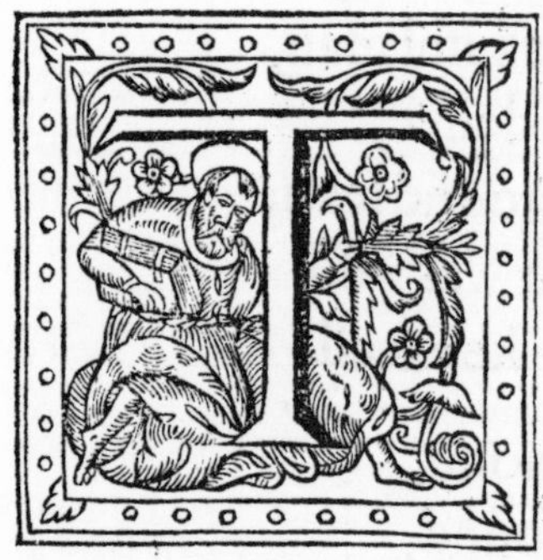

THE Diuine *Plato* in his Dialogue of health ſaith, that the controuerſies and diſputations of the writers doe open the truth. So is it at this time with many writers. For by their controuerſie in opinion, things are found out, which otherwiſe we would not haue looked for. And among all their controuerſies, I finde none more in doubt at this day, than is *Quickeſiluer*, which is moſt commonlie vſed about the curation of the diſeaſe called the *Frenchpocks*, for the opinion of the learned men are on both parts, and great reaſons the one againſt the other, that it makes many ſtand in doubt which ſide to take. Therefore at this preſent I haue taken in hand to write ſome proofes as concerning the properties of it, according to my ſimple knowledge: partly by the reading of Authors, and alſo as I haue found out by mine owne practiſe. But if thoſe learned men that haue written againſt it, did as well trie by practiſe as they do by their ſtudie to maintaine arguments, I thinke it would fall out that they would rather write in the defence of it: for I dare be bold to affirme, that ſome write more for arguments ſake, than for the truth, and other ſome for their vaine glory to be contrary to others, thinking therby to be counted the more famous.

Let them be neuer ſo well learned, that write of any thing, if I finde it otherwiſe by experience, and reaſon on my ſide too, I will prefer that before all others: for the truth ought to take place, and be preferred before their painted arguments: and for the truths ſake, I will write the profit that I haue found out by it.

And firſt I will ſhew the nature and propertie of the *Quickeſiluer*, for that is it that they all ſhoot at, *Marianus ſanctus Barolitanus*, a man of moſt excellent knowledge in the Art of Chirurgery, writing *De cauſa & defenſione*, making ſome digreſſion, ſaith, that he hath ſeene many which haue ſwallowed downe *Quickeſiluer* without any offence or harme, and for the confirmation of the ſame, he reciteth an hiſtory of a certaine woman, which at ſundry times tooke the quantitie of a

pound

pound and a halfe, which ſhee voided downward without any harme: more he ſaith, that many are deliuered from the *Iliaque paſſion* by the taking of it, which is a deadlie diſeaſe.

Auicen alſo approoueth in the Chapter *de Argento viuo*, that many haue taken it inwardly without any harme. Alſo *Antonius Muſa*, in his booke of ſimple medicines, and in his Treatiſe of metals, ſaith, that he did vſe to giue *Quickeſiluer* to children, being at the point of death through woormes. I my ſelfe to trie the truth, haue giuen it to many dogs, and other liuing things, which neuer had harme by it: whereof any man that doubteth may prooue.

Some ſay, that *Galen* affirmeth it to be venemous. *Galen* indeed in his ninth booke of Simples, confeſſeth that he neuer did experiment it. For whether it were taken in, or applied outwardly, he could not account it mortall. *Auicen* ordained it in his ointments for childrens ſore heads: and *Meſua* ordained it in his ointments for the ſcabs, in as great quantitie as we vſe it in any of our ointments.

All theſe authorities, who ſo liſt to read them, may plainly ſee that cruell qualitie, as ſome haue affirmed: and yet I will not ſay, but that through the vndiſcreet handling of it, many euils may happen, the which is not to be attributed to the thing, but to the worker. For what purging inward medicine haue you, but there is ſome venemous qualitie in it, and yet neuertheleſſe with their correctiues are ſo rectified from all their euill qualities, that they do their actions without any offence: for by the counſell of *Galen*, and all other ancient Authors, do we not vſe medicines inwardly, which be very venemous, as of Vipers, Hemlock, Henbane, Mandrake, Opium, Poppie, Helllebore, and others, the which may in ſuch ſort be corrected, that they may ſafely be taken inwardly without any harme?

Alſo many times through the vnskilfull handling of *Agaricke*, *Scammony*, *Turbit*, *Cartem*, yea & alſo *Rubarbe*, that are excellent purging medicines, (which men of knowledge vſe daily without harme) yet to many haue left ſuch a weakneſſe of the ſtomack, that there hath followed *Lienteria*, a continuall vomiting of the meate, by the which followed *Diſenteria*, *Tenaſmus*, and other ſuch accidents: And ſhall we condemne all thoſe good and wholeſome medicines, for the vndiſcreet handling of them? Let vs condemne bread and meate: for do we not ſee many a man die and periſh through the exceſſe of [illegible] As after any great famine we may ſee what harme doth come through the [illegible]ermuch taking of it, and yet meaſurably taken nothing more wholſom[illegible] nouriſhing.

And likewiſe of wine we see what euils do daily come by the vnmeaſurable taking of it. For beſides the euils that it brings to the liuer, it doth ſo coole and weaken the ſinewes, that commonly they fall to *Vertiginie*, *Scotomie*, *Apoplexie*, and ſo commonly death. No more reaſon is there to attribute the malice of the *Quckeſiluer*, vndiſcreetly handled, than there is to the others being of moſt wholſome qualities.

And now if you do not beleeue thoſe familiar examples, let vs come to the experience of it: I could bring foorth them that haue beene taken in hand of diuers for the ſame diſeaſe, and could neuer finde remedie by whatſoeuer they could do, which by the helpe of the ointment made with the ſaid *Quickeſiluer* being artificially handled, haue beene made perfectly well. Peraduenture you will obiect and ſay, that it is for a certaine time, and will returne afterwards.

To anſwere the which I will approoue, and not onely my ſelfe, but alſo many others of my company, Chirurgions in this City, that we haue cured a great number, which will confeſſe themſelues that they are as wel as euer they were in their liues. Which is eaſily knowen, for they are wel coloured, haue good appetite to eate, ſleepe well, & do al actions as well as euer they did in all their liues: and I wil affirme, that none of them being artificially cured, neuer haue fallen into the diſeaſe againe. Let vs therefore vſe that thing which is moſt manifeſtly approoued, and leaue the diſputation of ſuch as would make vs beleeue the things which are not. For (ſay they) it is cold, and through the coldneſſe of it, bringeth many euill accidents. Which is altogither falſe: for read *Galen*, in his fourth booke *De ſimplicibus*, and there you ſhall ſee the contrary.

Alſo read. *Ariſtoteles*. 4. *Meteor*, *Haliabas*, *Paule Ægineta*, *Conſtantine*, *Iſaac*, *Raſſius*, *Platerius*, & yee ſhall be fully ſatisfied. And if theſe Authors will not perſwade, let experience teach: for it doth extenuate and reſolue, which both are actions of heate, and not of cold. The reaſon which they yeelde that it is cold, is bicauſe it is made of Lead. Which followeth not: for we ſee that Lime is made of Chalke, which is a cold ſtone, and yet the Lime is hot. Diuers other examples I could bring in, for the proofe of that, which for breuity ſake I will let paſſe, referring the indifferent reader to others, which haue written of this matter.

Among the reſt, this booke for the true practiſe, I thinke to be one of the cheifeſt that hath beene publiſhed in our tong, [illegible] now the third time corrected, and inlarged, wherein [illegible] beene taken great paines, for the which we deſire [illegible] but good ſpeeches: though that ſome of late haue rewarded both of vs with euill words,

and

and alſo ſought to deface our writings, if their wil and their wit could haue agreed.

But this we would haue knowen vnto them, that there is neither of vs both, but haue cured more in number, than euer they did ſee in all their liues, that hath moſt found fault with our writings, and are able to prooue by reaſon our doings therein. I thinke rather it was for enuie, than for any zeale to the truth of the matter: being not wel contented to ſee others in better credite and doings than themſelues.

Let them not malice vs: for it is the good liking of the people, in that we haue diſcharged our duties. It may be, that when they haue practiſed ſo long in this Citie, and other places of this Realme as we haue done, they may haue as good dooings as we haue, if they diſcharge their duties accordingly: if not, let them be ſure, the longer they practiſe, the woorſe it will be for them, the which we would be loth to ſee. For it is the comfort of euery honeſt Artiſt, to ſee the profeſſors to floriſh, and eſpecially being of one body and company, for one member not doing his duty, all the reſt fare the woorſe: therefore, we ſhould rather be a comfort the one to the other, than to deface one anothers doings.

I would to God, that it were well conſidered of vs, and that there might be an vnion among vs which profeſſe this noble Art of Chirurgery, that we may diſcharge our duties in the common wealth, to the glory of God, and the one to be a helpe and comfort to the other.

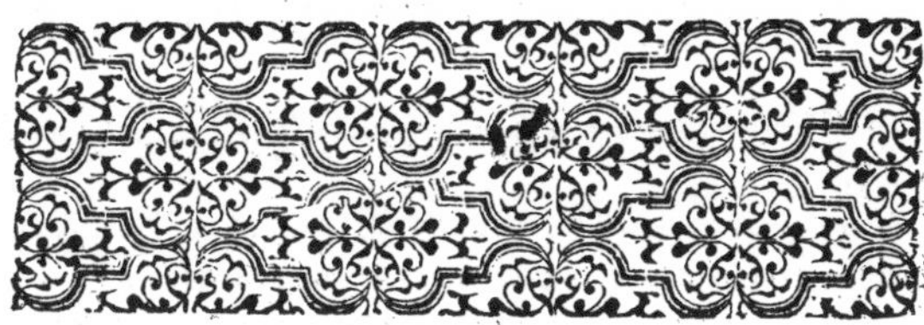

THE TABLE.

The

Of

The Table.

FINIS.